PLANT-BASED DIET COOKBOOK:
THE COMPLETE GUIDE FOR BEGINNERS WITH DELICIOUS RECIPES AND MEAL PLAN.

Table of Contents

Introduction

A plant-based diet is a diet that is based primarily on whole plant foods. It is identical to the regular diet we're used to already, except that it leaves out foods not exclusively from plants. Hence, a plant-based diet does away with all types of animal-sourced foods, hydrogenated oils, refined sugars, and processed foods. Instead, a whole food plant-based diet comprises fruits and vegetables and unprocessed or barely-processed oils with healthy monounsaturated fats (like extra-virgin olive oil), whole grains, and legumes (essentially lentils and beans).

A plant-based diet is a diet that has roots in the traditional diets of our ancestors, and it is also how most cultures around the world eat. Many present-day diseases such as cancer, heart disease, or diabetes can often be directly linked to the typical Western diet.

A plant-based diet embraces food as a powerful tool for health and wellness. Eating more unprocessed whole foods can go a long way to reduce the risk of chronic diseases and improve overall well-being and vitality. It can also help fight many serious diseases such as diabetes and heart disease, which we hear about every day in the news.

It is interesting to note that many scientists use the word "vegan" instead of "plant-based," which implies that they define vegans as people who avoid all types of animal-sourced foods for ethical reasons. These so-called "vegans" are still eating animal products because they do not avoid them just because they are animals or because there is no other reasonable way to obtain them. Many vegans also fall into the trap of consuming refined sugars and processed foods just because these items are readily available. A plant-based diet, however, is much more than just veganism.

A plant-based diet has very few limitations. It leaves absolutely no room for junk foods or refined sugars, or processed foods. It can be broken down into three main food groups: fruits, vegetables and whole grains, legumes, and beans. This way of eating is healthy enough to be followed for life.

The advantages of following a plant-based diet are many. First, for your overall health, it is the best thing you can do because it greatly reduces the possibility of developing certain types of cancers (such as the colon), heart disease (in particular heart attacks), diabetes (type II), or strokes. It will even help lower the risk of death from many other diseases, such as Parkinson's disease, Alzheimer's disease, and even numerous types of cancer.

A plant-based diet is very simple and does not require a lot of time and effort to prepare. It can be done during lunchtime, which gives you an extra hour of free time each day, and it can also be done during the weekend; it's up to you. You will need to make minor changes in the kitchen, such as buying different oils (I like olive oil), but it's already there. Many of us are used to eating polished,

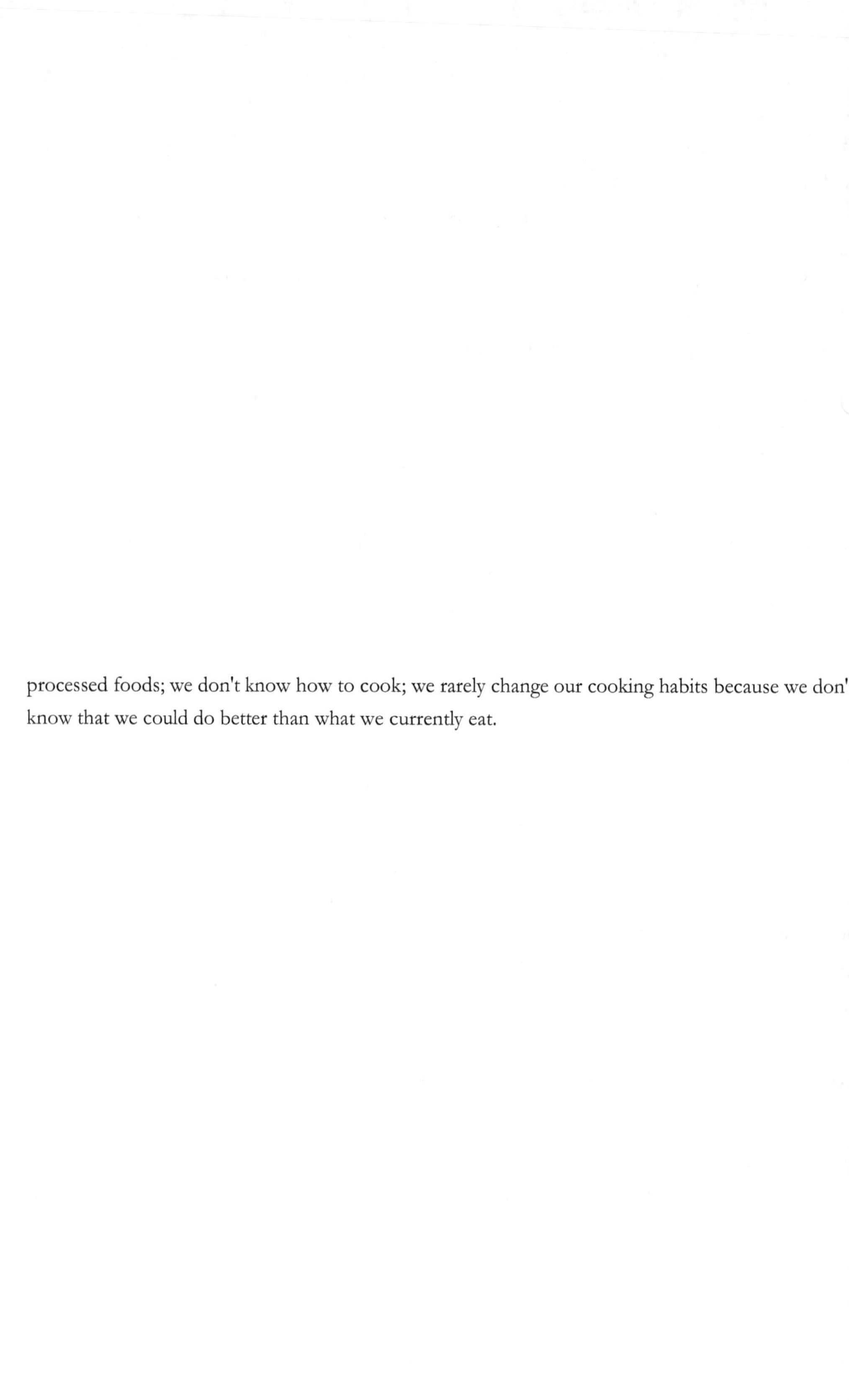

processed foods; we don't know how to cook; we rarely change our cooking habits because we don't know that we could do better than what we currently eat.

Chapter 1.   What is a plant-based diet?

A plant-based diet is more of a way of eating foods made by nature. This diet is based on fruits, vegetables, whole grains, legumes, nuts, seeds, herbs, roots, sweeteners, oils, and beverages. These are all foods that are, in one way or another, directly derived from plants. Scientific studies have proven that people following plant-based diets are generally healthier than others. Many of these foods are also environmentally friendlier than the kinds of foods we've been eating for the past several thousands of years. Nowadays, following this lifestyle is also easier because of the many plant-based products available at the grocery store, but it does require some knowledge on nutrition, eating, and cooking.

The reason why this diet is called plant-based is because it is very much the same as humans eating whole plant foods. Nowadays, people often chose to eat animal-based foods because there are many ways to enhance the taste of these foods, because they come in a more convenient form, and because these foods offer a different kind of nutritional value. This lifestyle requires a lot of knowledge on food, eating, and cooking. It is a "clean eating" lifestyle, and it involves a big change from the whole foods diet that the average person following the Standard American Diet follows. In the plant-based diet, all meals are composed of whole plant foods. This means no refined sugar or flours, no processed or packaged or fast foods, no oils that are usually used in cooking, and no animal-based foods.

This diet offers a whole lot of health benefits. It is very effective in weight management, diabetes management, lowering one's blood cholesterol level, strengthening the immune system, maintaining healthy eating habits, preventing certain lifestyle-related diseases, improving digestive function, promoting healthy living, and eliminating animal-based foods.

In general, the plant-based diet is healthy, nutritious, and full of life giving whole foods. However, some foods that are more processed and made from a mixture of raw and dry beans, seeds, and grains do have a high amount of nutritional value. Eating a vegetable diet is a great way to get a lot of the nutrients that you need. Most plant-based diets include a lot of fruit, vegetables, whole grains, legumes, nuts, and seeds.

In general, following a plant-based diet will promote a lot of health benefits.

An herbivorous diet is primarily based on plants for food, in contrast to diets based on meat, eggs or dairy products. This encompasses a wide variety of plant-based diets, incorporating all types of fruits, vegetables, nuts, seeds, grains and plants eaten in any quantity for the primary purpose of nourishment.

Chapter 2.   Benefits of Plant-based Diet

In recent years, a huge surge of people has been taking up a plant-based diet as a lifestyle choice. In recent times, a lot of studies have been conducted on the topic of a plant-based diet's effects on health. There have been studies that have shown positive health effects of a plant-based diet.

A plant-based diet consists of a lot of vegetables and a small amount of fruit; that's why it's referred to as a food-based diet.

This diet is typically low in fat, sodium, and cholesterol. It is high in fiber, vitamins, and minerals that are beneficial to health.

It is high in antioxidants that can reduce cancer risk and oxidative stress. A plant-based diet had shown to help lower the risk of heart disease, type-2 diabetes, strokes, and several types of cancer.

A plant-based diet that is rich in fiber has also been shown to help keep you full. Research shows that the intake of fruits and vegetables can reduce your chances of developing type-2 diabetes by up to 25 percent.

Through the consumption of plant-based foods, you get the nutrients you need to stay healthy. Plant-based foods include fresh fruits, vegetables, whole grains, legumes, nuts, and seeds.

Plant-based foods are devoid of saturated fats, are high in fiber, are low in calories, are rich in nutrients, are more easily digested by the body, are absolutely beneficial for health, are full of antioxidants, are easy on your digestive system, are anti-inflammatory, are more easily broken down by the body.

Plant-based foods are low in calories, and this allows an individual to eat more of the same while staying fit.

Plant-based foods aid the individual against all diseases and maintain a healthy lifestyle. Because plant-based foods aid against all diseases, a plant-based diet can be a lifetime cure for heart disease, diabetes, obesity, etc.

Plant-based foods such as fruits, whole grains, vegetables, legumes, nuts, and seeds contain fiber that fills you up, gives you a feeling of fullness and eliminates cravings. Plant foods provide more than the required energy and nutrients and eliminate the need for refined sugars and all kinds of processed foods and junk foods.

The best thing about a plant-based diet is that it's virtually devoid of saturated fats and refined sugars, and junk foods. Contrary to popular belief, substituting animal protein with plant protein is not good for health.

Plant foods are the foods on earth that are made of the most naked amino acids, where protein is found. Plant protein is also high in immune-boosting antioxidants, which are very good for health. Plant protein is absolutely free of any allergens and is easily digested.

In a plant-based diet, different foods can be combined while trying to get a variety of nutrients, exactly like with a variety of fruits and vegetables. This is why adopting a plant-based diet is such a great idea.

Chapter 3.   Food to eat and what not to eat on a plant-based diet

This diet is a good choice for anyone interested in healthy living. A plant-based diet disregards all animal products, including meat, dairy, seafood, and eggs. It's also called a vegan diet or veganism. A vegan diet allows you to consume foods that are rich in nutrients and maximize your health benefits.

Food to eat

In this book, I will briefly cover the top 10 best foods to eat on a plant-based diet.

Here we go:

1. Fruit and vegetables

Fruits and vegetables are the healthiest food you can eat on a vegan diet. They're high in fiber, vitamins, minerals, and antioxidants.

2. Beans

Beans are another excellent food to eat on a vegan diet. They are not only high in fiber but also rich in protein, magnesium, and B vitamins. Beans also keep you full for a longer period of time without the need for added fat and calories.

3. Whole Grains

It is rich in   minerals, and B vitamins. Grains are rich in antioxidants, which help lower your risk of having certain diseases like heart disease, diabetes, and cancer.

4. Nuts and Seeds

Nuts and seeds are great for snacking. They're rich in healthy fats, protein, and fiber. These little gems also contain healthy plant oils that help lower bad LDL cholesterol levels

5. Whole Wheat Couscous

Whole wheat couscous contains all the essential amino acids, vitamins, and minerals you need to lead an active lifestyle. Couscous is also high in fiber. If you're on a vegan diet and finding it difficult to get enough protein, couscous is a great alternative to meat.

6. Hemp Seeds

Hemp seeds, or ground hemp seeds, are a good source of protein and essential fatty acids. This little gem packs a ton of nutritional punch without any cholesterol or saturated fat. Add hemp seeds to your favorite salad for more flavor and crunch. Hemp seeds also make a delicious topping for your morning cereal or yogurt.

7. Spirulina

Spirulina is a sea-based plant that has been around for over 3 billion years. It's filled with protein and B vitamins, and antioxidants that help your body lower blood sugar levels and increase your energy levels.

8. Hemp Milk

Hemp milk is rich in "good" fats omega-3 and omega-6, zinc, and protein. It's also cholesterol-free! Use hemp milk in place of regular milk when cooking or drinking cereal or coffee in the morning for a delicious, healthy treat.

9. Chia Seeds

Ground chia seeds are high in protein, antioxidants, and essential fatty acids. Chia seeds are great for snacking on or adding to your favorite smoothie.

10. Flaxseeds

Flaxseeds help you lower your risk of heart disease, diabetes, cancer, obesity, and depression. They're one of the best healthy living foods out there. Flaxseeds can be added to yogurt or cereal for a healthy start to your day. Mix ground flax into your smoothies for an added nutritional punch, or sprinkle them on salads or soup for added flavor.

What not to eat on a plant-based diet

A plant-based diet is good for both the body and mind because it clears out toxins, which can lead to enhanced brain function, and it is good for the environment because animal agriculture contributes to the destruction of many types of plants and animals around the world.

There are certain foods that must be avoided on a plant-based diet. Plant-based diets shouldn't be eating anything with meat or any meat-like substance. Here is a food list that you should not eat if you want to follow a plant-based diet.

- Meat
- Soy
- Soybeans
- Bean curd
- Bean sprouts
- Grains
- Dairy

- Eggs
- Poultry
- Fish

1. Meat

Let us start from meat because it is one of the worst additions to a diet that seeks a healthy planet.

There are many things wrong with eating meat. Firstly, it's that the process in which animals are mass-produced for consumption causes a great deal of environmental pollution.

Given this, it is no surprise that meat is consistently ranked as one of the worst things one can eat on a plant-based diet.

2. Soy

Soy is a good source of protein because it contains protease inhibitors, but it is best avoided on a plant-based diet.

Firstly, soy is often genetically modified. Genetically modifying food items deprives people of their own decision on what they are eating. Genetically modified ingredients in foods are increasingly common and cause many different adverse health effects, including infertility in females and an increased risk of cancer in men.

Secondly, soy does not provide nutritional value. It often actually detracts from nutrition. Soy is an inefficient source of nutrients because it doesn't provide easily digestible proteins (abstaining from beef helps ensure you don't need to worry about this).

Thirdly, soy is overly processed, and it can't be good for our digestive system. Soybeans are poorly digested by the human body and contain phytic acid (the same substance that can cause digestive problems for people who eat lots of grains, like rice).

So how do you know, if you've abstained from soy, that it won't cause you gastrointestinal problems? Simple. Soy is a common allergen.

3. Grains

Grains are not a healthy addition to a plant-based diet. Grains are not even plant-based, but grains consist of seeds from plants, which are not plants.

Grains provide a satisfying amount of energy. They are very good for people who need a ton of energy because they give a lot of energy, especially carbohydrates. However, there are many bad things about grains that outweigh the benefits.

Firstly, grains are often processed. There are many examples of foods made out of grains, which are not as helpful as they should be. When grains are harvested, the grains are ground and mixed with other powerful things (like sugar and oil) to make lots of products. Just as with any food product, over-processed foods have a high risk of being unhealthy.

Secondly, grains, being a type of seed, cause allergic reactions. This is another thing that is common with grains, and wheat is particularly problematic for this.

Thirdly, grains, in general, are terrible for soil health. They aren't very great for the soil because they can't be digested, and compaction is a major factor in the compaction of soil, which can lead to soil degradation.

4. Bean curd

Bean curd is something that people want to eat because it is tasty, but it is not that great for eating. Bean curd is the tofu that people try to say tastes good. It can be eaten as a whole, as a bean curd patty, or as a pizza topping.

Bean curd is problematic for eating from a plant-based diet. Why?

Bean curd contains lysine monochlorohydrochloride. Lysine monochlorohydrochloride can cause severe kidney damage if ingested regularly. It can cause these side effects because it is classified as a toxic substance. It is used for industrial purposes and has been deemed harmful to humans.

So if you want to stay away from a world of possible kidney failure, it's a good idea to stay away from bean curd.

5. Bean sprouts

Bean sprouts are another food that people don't expect to have a plant-based alternative for. Bean sprouts are the young plants of beans. They're also very good for eating.

However, bean sprouts contain a toxic plant chemical called benzyl cyanide. When it is consumed, it actually builds up in the human body and makes you more and more susceptible to kidney and liver damage.

There is a way to avoid it, and that is to boil bean sprouts. This almost completely kills most of the benzyl cyanide. However, it's best to just avoid bean sprouts completely, just to be safe.

6. Dairy

Dairy has a lot of great things, especially about it, but there is a common myth about dairy. It is believed that dairy products contain calcium and protein, and they do. However, these two things aren't the best sources of protein and calcium.

Dairy products contain a lot of fat. A lot of fat can result in cholesterol showing up in the blood. Blood cholesterol is the main cause of strokes and heart attacks.

7. Beef

Beef is very bad for us. It is the most disease-ridden food in the world (compared to chicken and pork, anyway). Why?

Firstly, beef is the only source of Mad Cow Disease. Mad Cow Disease is a brain disease that causes mental disabilities. Cerebellar ataxia is the main symptom.

Secondly, another dangerous disease can be contracted by eating beef. It is called bovine spongiform encephalopathy. This is the same disease that causes Mad Cow Disease. It causes brain damage, or spongiform encephalopathy, in the brain.

Were this all the bad stuff, you should probably avoid it. You could also lower your risk of illnesses by eating more plant-based food.

Chapter 4.   Breakfast

1. Avocado Toast with White Beans

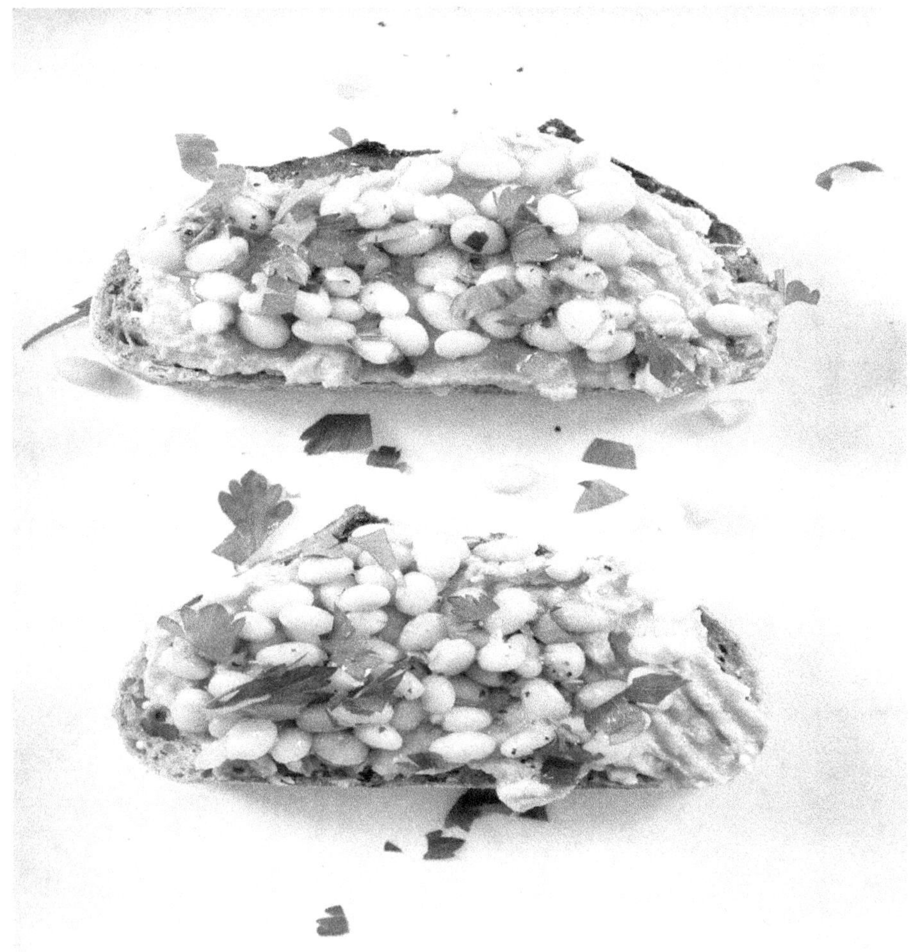

Preparation Time: 5 minutes

Cooking Time: 6 minutes

Servings: 4

Ingredients:

- ½ cup canned white beans, drained and rinsed
- 2 teaspoons tahini paste
- 2 teaspoons lemon juice
- ½ teaspoon salt

- ½ avocado, peeled and pit removed
- 4 slices whole-grain bread, toasted
- ½ cup grape tomatoes, cut in half

Directions:

1. Grab a small bowl and add the beans, tahini, ½ the lemon juice, and ½ the salt. Mash with a fork.
2. Take another bowl and add the avocado and the remaining lemon juice and salt. Mash together.
3. Place your toast onto a flat surface and add the mashed beans, spreading well.
4. Top with the avocado and the sliced tomatoes then serve and enjoy.

Nutrition:

Calories 140

Fat 5

Carbs 13

Protein 5

2. Oatmeal & Peanut Butter Breakfast Bar

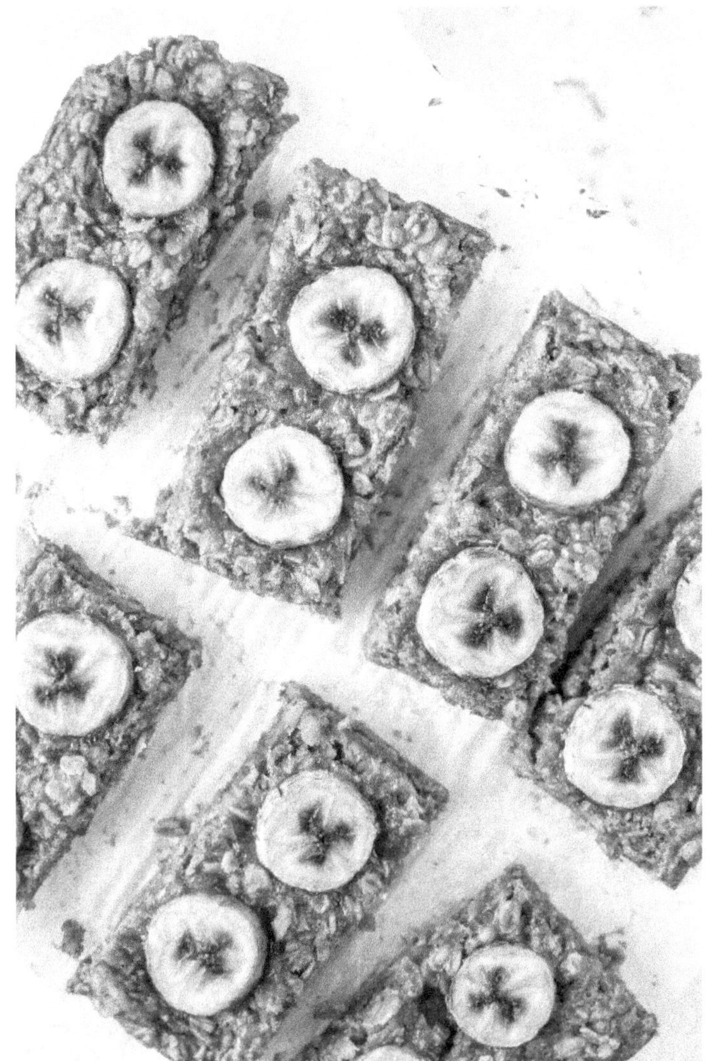

Preparation Time: 10 minutes

Cooking Time: 0 minutes

Servings: 8

Ingredients:

- 1 ½ cups date, pit removed
- ½ cup peanut butter
- ½ cup old-fashioned rolled oats

Directions:

1. Grease a baking tin and pop to one side.

2. Grab your food processor, add the dates, and whizz until chopped.

3. Add the peanut butter and the oats and pulse.

4. Scoop into the baking tin then pop into the fridge or freezer until set.

5. Serve and enjoy.

Nutrition:

Calories 232

Fat 9

Carbs 32

Protein 8

3. Chocolate Chip Banana Pancake

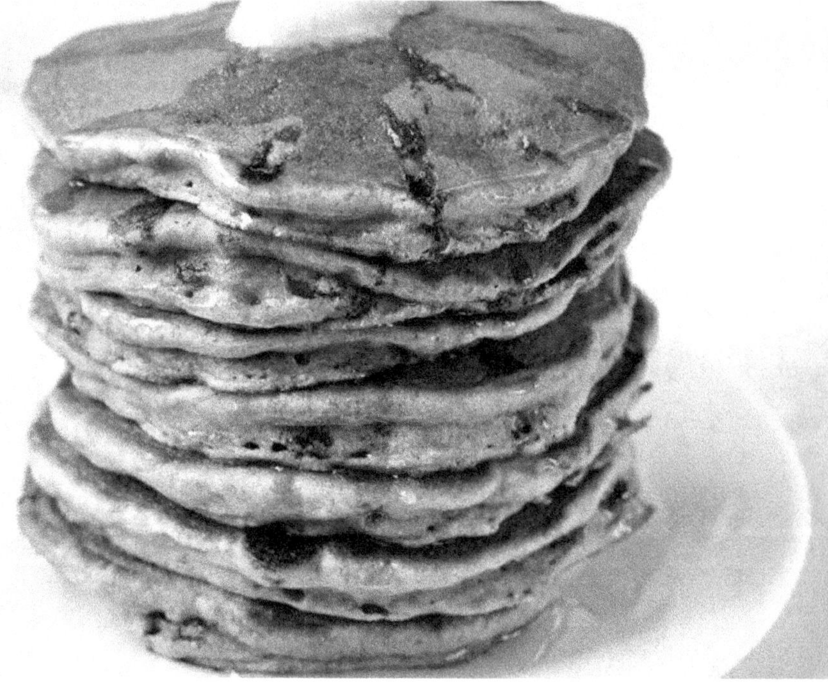

Preparation Time: 15 minutes

Cooking Time: 3 minutes

Servings: 6

Ingredients:

- 1 large ripe banana, mashed
- 2 tablespoons coconut sugar
- 3 tablespoons coconut oil, melted
- 1 cup of coconut milk
- 1 ½ cups whole wheat flour
- 1 teaspoon baking soda
- ½ cup vegan chocolate chips
- Olive oil, for frying

Directions:

1. Grab a large bowl and add the banana, sugar, oil, and milk. Stir well.
2. Add the flour and baking soda and stir again until combined.
3. Add the chocolate chips and fold through then pop to one side.
4. Put a skillet over medium heat and add a drop of oil.
5. Pour ¼ of the batter into the pan and move the pan to cover.
6. Cook for 3 minutes then flip and cook on the other side.
7. Repeat with the remaining pancakes then serve and enjoy.

Nutrition:

Calories 105

Fat 13

Carbs 23

Protein 5

4. Avocado and 'Sausage' Breakfast Sandwich

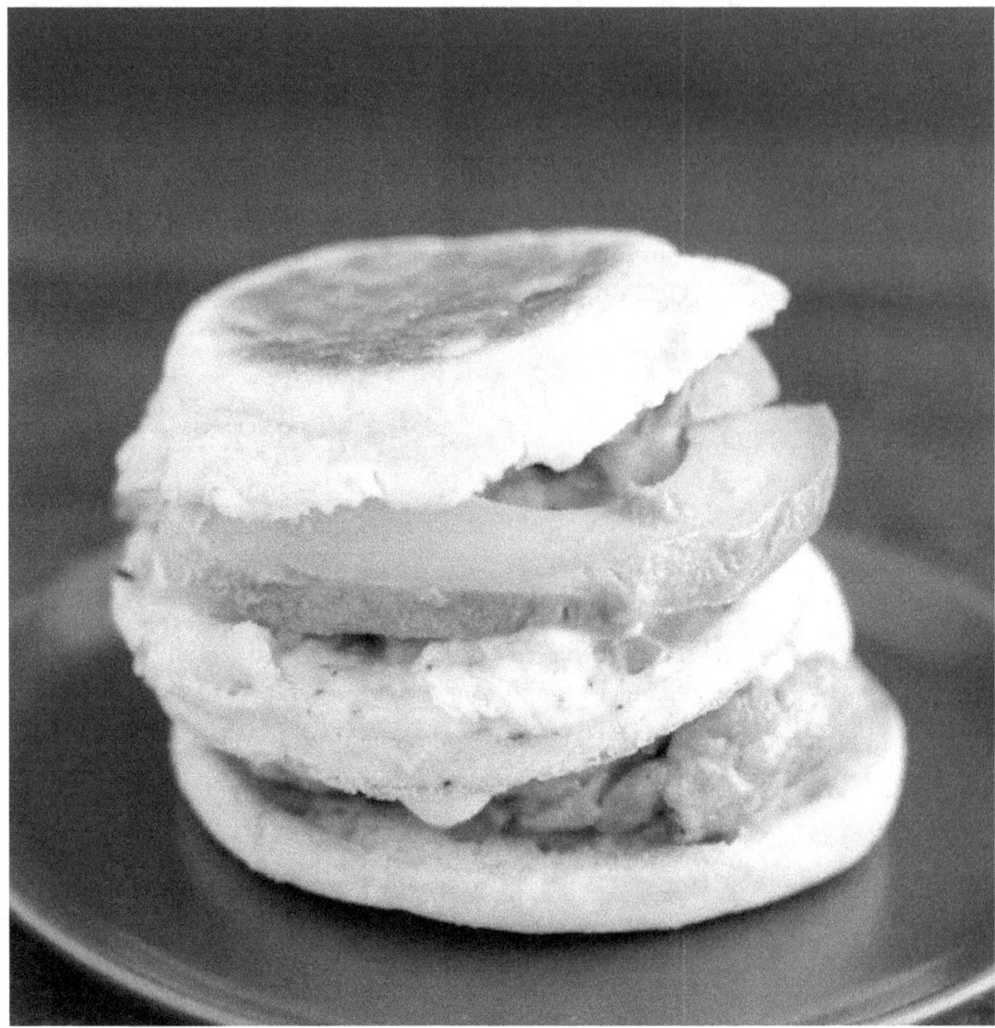

Preparation Time: 15 minutes

Cooking Time: 10 minutes

Servings: 1

Ingredients:

- 1 vegan sausage patty
- 1 cup kale, chopped
- 2 teaspoons extra virgin olive oil
- 1 tablespoon pepitas

- Salt and pepper, to taste
- 1 tablespoon vegan mayo
- 1/8 teaspoon chipotle powder
- 1 teaspoon jalapeno chopped
- 1 English muffin, toasted
- ¼ avocado, sliced

Directions:

1. Place a pan over heat and add a drop of oil.
2. Add the vegan patty and cook for 2 minutes.
3. Flip the patty then add the kale and pepitas.
4. Season well then cook for another few minutes until the patty is cooked.
5. Find a small bowl and add the mayo, chipotle powder, and the jalapeno. Stir well to combine.
6. Place the muffin onto a flat surface, spread with the spicy mayo then top with the patty.
7. Add the sliced avocado then serve and enjoy.

Nutrition:

Calories 573

Fat 23

Carbs 36

Protein 21

5. Vegan Variety Poppy Seed Scones

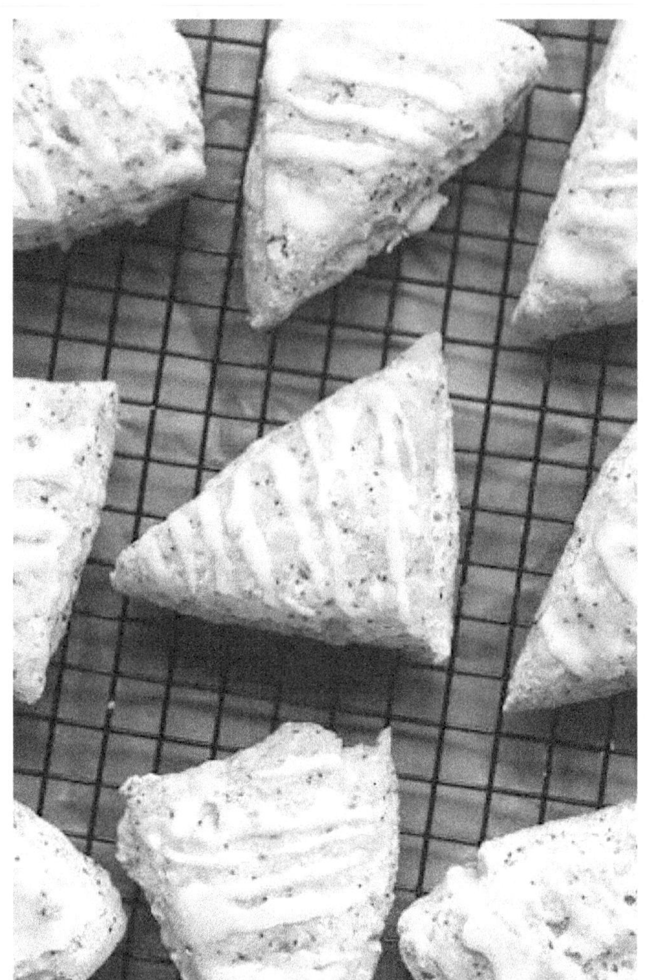

Preparation Time: 5 minutes

Cooking Time: 10 minutes

Servings: 12.

Ingredients:

- 1 cup white sugar
- 2 cups flour
- Juice from 1 lemon
- Zest from 1 lemon
- 4 teaspoon baking powder
- ½ teaspoon salt
- 1 cup Earth Balance or vegan butter
- 2 tablespoon poppy seeds

- ½ cup soymilk
- 1/3 cup water

Directions:

1. Start by heating the oven to 400 degrees Fahrenheit.
2. Next, mix the sugar, the flour, the powder, and the salt in a big mixing bowl. Add the vegan butter to the mixture and cut it up until you create a sand-like mixture. Next, add the lemon juice, the lemon zest, and the poppy seeds. Add the water and the soy milk, and stir the ingredients well.
3. Portion the batter out over a baking sheet in about ¼ cup portions. Allow the scones to bake for fifteen minutes and let them cool before serving. Enjoy.

Nutrition:

Calories 205

Fat 3

Carbs 12

Protein 6

6. Sweet Pomegranate Porridge

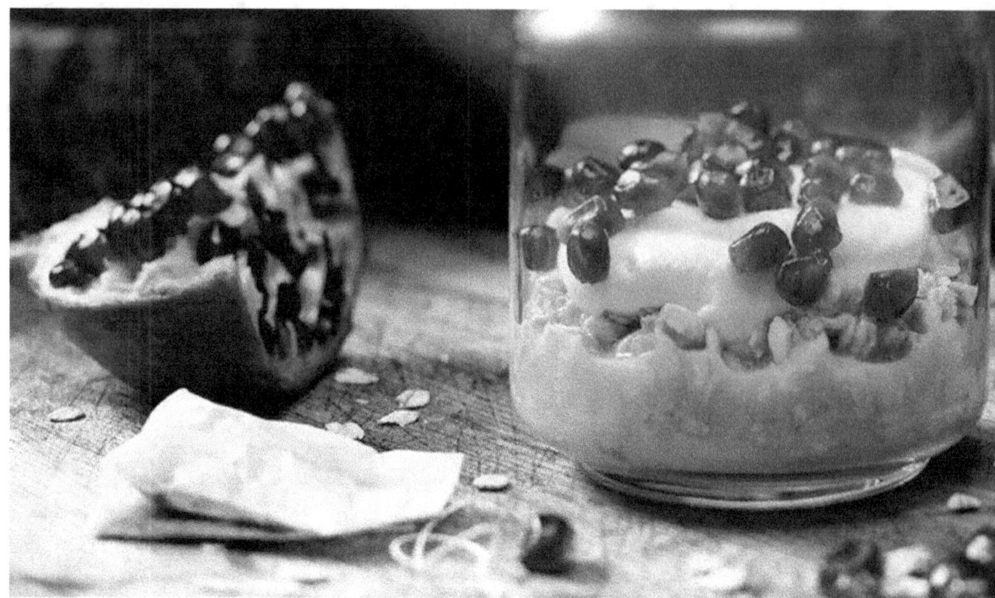

Preparation Time: 5 minutes

Cooking Time: 20 minutes

Servings: 4

Ingredients:

- 2 Cups Oats
- 1 ½ Cups Water
- 1 ½ Cups Pomegranate Juice
- 2 Tablespoons Pomegranate Molasses

Directions:

1. Empty all fixings into the instant pot and mix well.
2. Seal the lid, and cook on high pressure for four minutes.
3. Use a quick release, and serve warm.

Nutrition:

Calories 177

Fat 6

Carbs 23

7. Apple Oatmeal

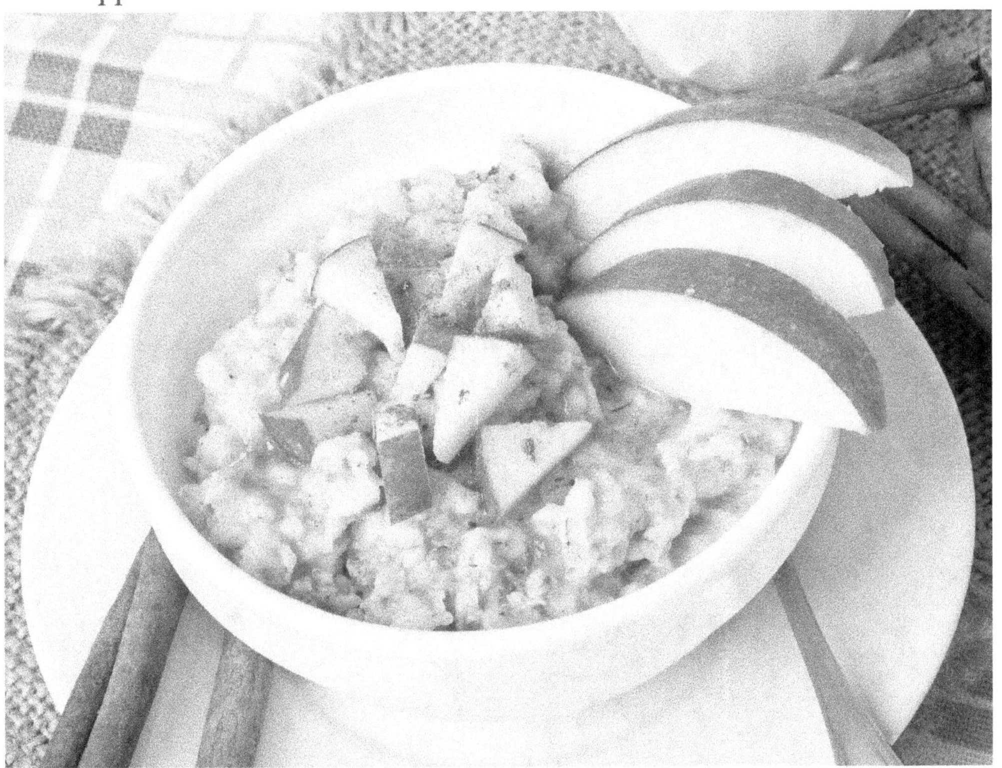

Preparation Time: 5 minutes

Cooking Time: 20 minutes

Servings: 4

Ingredients:

- ¼ Teaspoon Sea Salt
- 1 Cup Cashew Milk
- 1 Cup Strawberries, Halved & Fresh
- 1 Tablespoon Brown Sugar
- 2 Cups Apples, Diced
- 3 Cups Water
- ¼ Teaspoon Coconut Oil

- ½ Cup Steel Cut Oats

Directions:

1. Start by greasing your instant pot with oil, and add everything to it except for the milk and berries.
2. Cook on high pressure for ten minutes, and then add in your milk and strawberries. Mix well, and serve warm.

Nutrition:

Calories 435

Fat 7

Carbs 34

Protein 8

8. Vegan Breakfast Biscuits

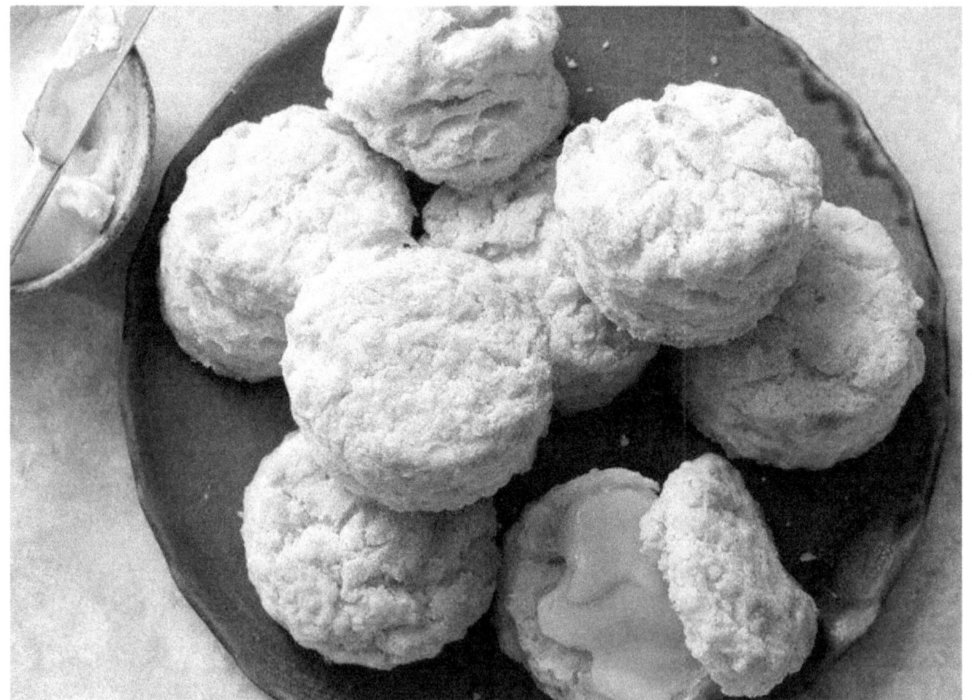

Preparation Time: 10 minutes

Cooking Time: 10 min

Servings: 6

Ingredients:

- cups Almond Flour   - quantity not mentioned
- 1 tbsp Baking Powder
- ¼ teaspoon Salt
- ½ teaspoon Onion Powder
- ½ cup Coconut Milk
- ¼ cup Nutritional Yeast
- 2 tbsp Ground Flax Seeds
- ¼ cup Olive Oil

Directions:

1. Preheat oven to 450F.
2. Whisk together all ingredients in a bowl.
3. Divide the batter into a pre-greased muffin tin.
4. Bake for 10 minutes.

Nutrition:

Calories 432

Fat 5

Carbs 13

Protein 8

Chapter 5.   Lunch

9. Chickpea Sunflower Sandwich

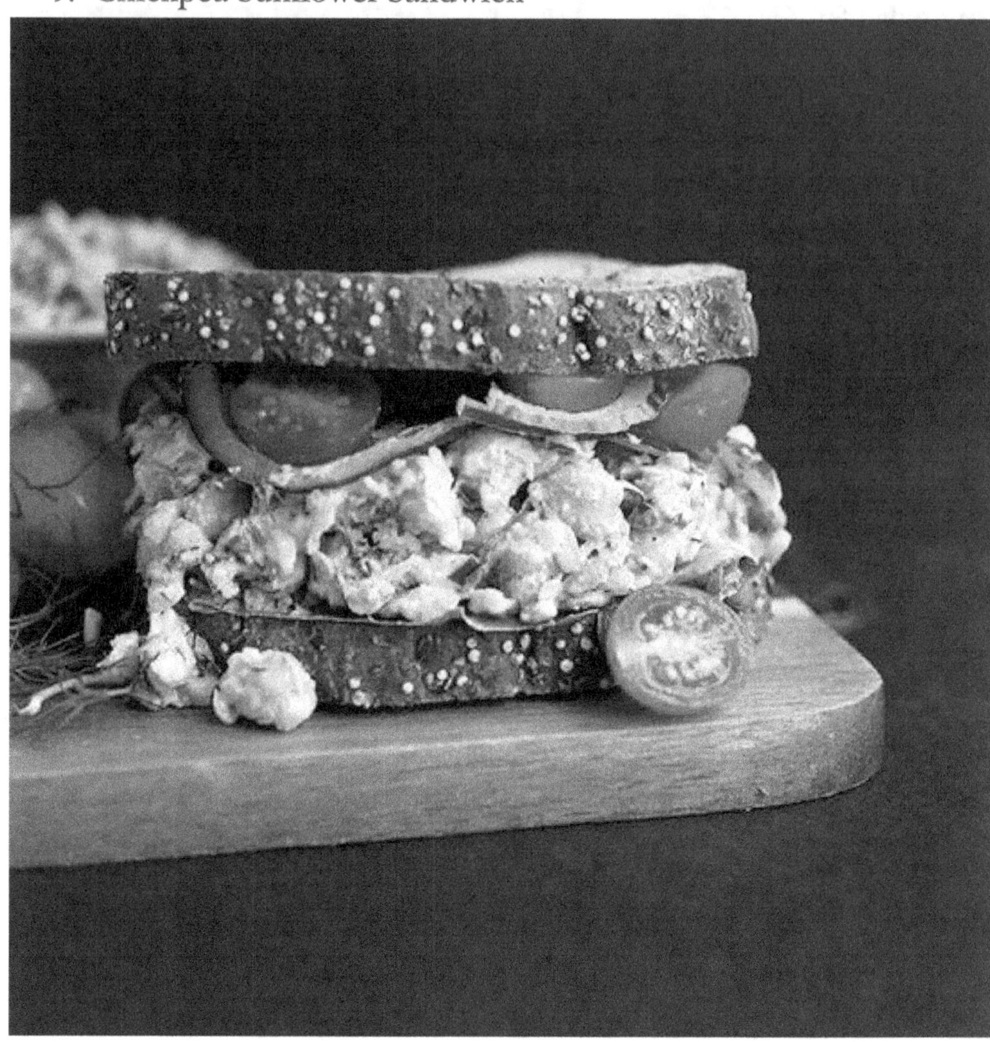

Preparation Time: 15 minutes

Cooking Time: 10 minutes

Servings: 2

Ingredients:

For The Sandwich:

- 1 ¾ cup cooked chickpeas
- 1/4 cup chopped red onion

- 1/4 cup roasted sunflower seeds, unsalted
- ½ teaspoon salt
- ¼ teaspoon ground black pepper
- 1 tablespoon maple syrup
- 1/2 teaspoon Dijon mustard
- 3 tablespoons vegan mayonnaise
- 2 tablespoons fresh dill
- 4 pieces of rustic bread

For The Garlic Herb Sauce:

- 1 teaspoon minced garlic
- 1/2 of lemon, juiced
- ½ teaspoon of sea salt
- 1 teaspoon dried dill
- ¼ dried dill
- 1/4 cup hummus
- ¼ cup almond milk, unsweetened

For Topping:

- 1 avocado, pitted, sliced
- 1 medium white onion, peeled, sliced
- ½ cup chopped lettuce
- 1 medium tomato, sliced

Directions:

1. Prepare the garlic herb sauce and for this, take a medium bowl, place all of its fixings and whisk until combined, set aside until combined.
2. Take a medium bowl, add chickpeas in it, and then mash by using a fork until broken.
3. Then add onion, dill, sunflower seeds, salt, black pepper, mustard, maple syrup, and mayonnaise and stir until well combined.
4. Take a medium skillet pan, place it over medium heat, add bread slices, and cook for 3 minutes per side until toasted.
5. Spread chickpea mixture on one side of two bread slices, top with prepared garlic herb sauce, avocado, onion, tomato, and lettuce and cover with the other two slices.
6. Serve straight away.

Nutrition:

532 Cal

30 g Fat

4 g Saturated Fat

52 g Carbohydrates

14 g Fiber

8 g Sugars

17 g Protein;

10. White Bean and Artichoke Sandwich

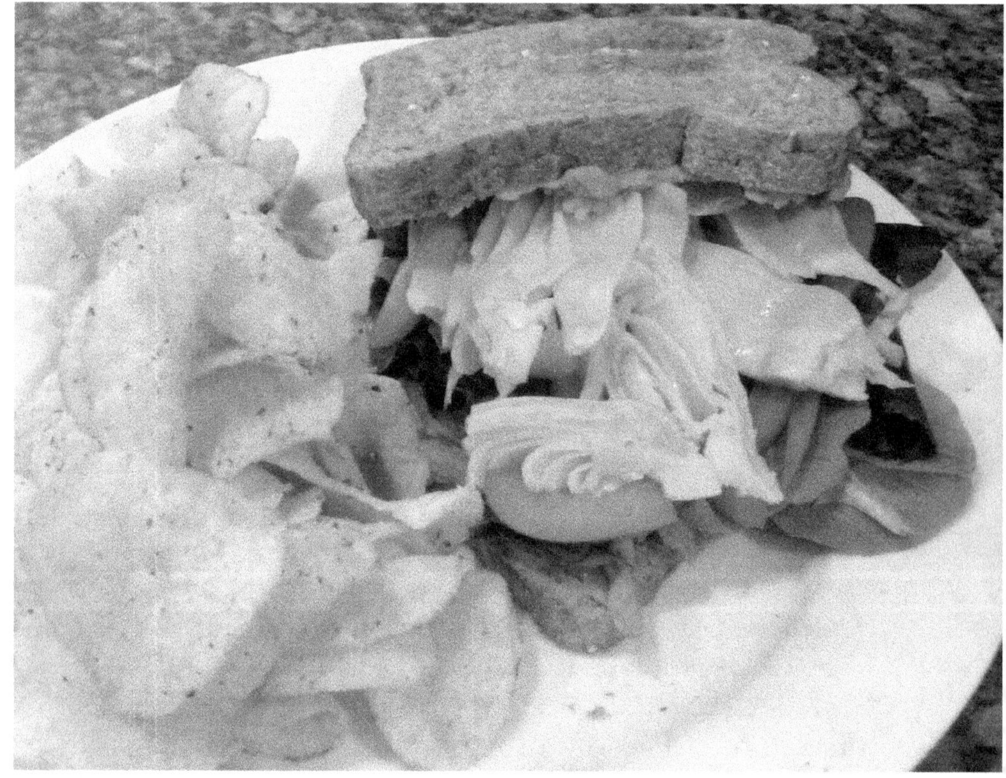

nPreparation Time: 15 minutes

Cooking Time: 10 minutes

Servings: 4

Ingredients:

- 1 ¼ cooked white beans
- ½ cup cashew nuts
- 6 artichoke hearts, chopped
- ¼ cup sunflower seeds, hulled
- 1 clove of garlic, peeled
- ¼ teaspoon salt
- ¼ teaspoon ground black pepper
- 1 teaspoon dried rosemary
- 1 lemon, grated
- 6 tablespoons almond milk, unsweetened
- 8 pieces of rustic bread

Directions:

1. Immerse cashew nuts in warm water for 10 minutes, then drain them and transfer into a food processor.
2. Add garlic, salt, black pepper, rosemary, lemon zest, and milk and then pulse for 2 minutes.
3. Take a medium bowl, place beans in it, mash them by using a fork, then add sunflower seeds and artichokes and stir until mixed.
4. Pour in cashew nuts dressing, stir until coated, and taste to adjust seasoning.
5. Take a medium skillet pan, place it over medium heat, add bread slices, and cook for 3 minutes per side until toasted.
6. Spread white beans mixture on one side of four bread slices and then cover with the other four slices.
7. Serve straight away.

Nutrition:

220 Cal

8 g Fat

1 g Saturated Fat

28 g Carbohydrates

8 g Fiber

2 g Sugars

12 g Protein;

11. Egg Salad Sandwich

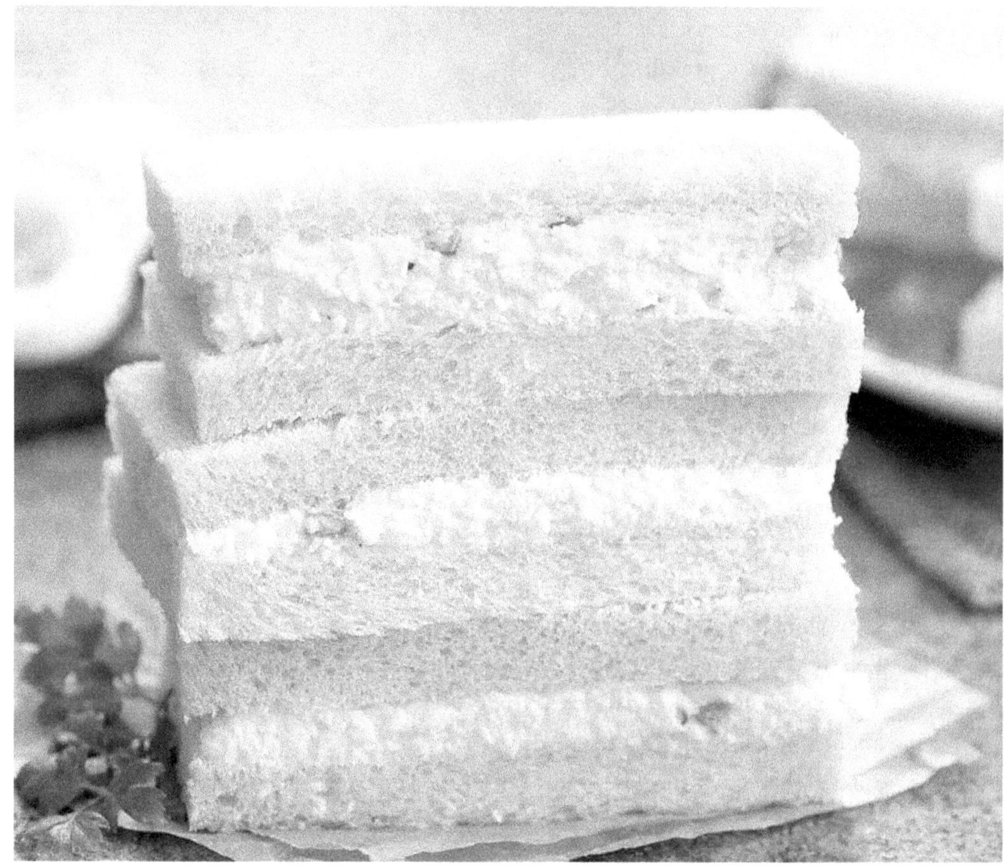

Preparation Time: 5 minutes

Cooking Time: 0 minutes

Servings: 4

Ingredients:

- 12 ounces tofu, extra-firm, pressed, drained
- 4 tablespoon sliced green onion

- ¼ teaspoon ground black pepper
- ½ teaspoon black salt
- 1/8 teaspoon turmeric powder
- 1 teaspoon mustard powder
- 8 teaspoons pumpkin seeds, shelled
- 4 tablespoon mayonnaise
- 8 slices of sandwich bread

Directions:

1. Take a medium bowl, place tofu in it, and then crumble it by using fingers.
2. Add remaining ingredients except for bread and stir until well combined, taste to adjust seasoning.
3. Take a medium skillet pan, place it over medium heat, add bread slices, and cook for 3 minutes per side until toasted.
4. Spread tofu mixture on one side of four bread slices and then cover with the other four slices.
5. Serve straight away.

Nutrition:

347 Cal

17 g Fat

2 g Saturated Fat

32 g Carbohydrates

2 g Fiber

4 g Sugars

15 g Protein;

12. Sabich Sandwich

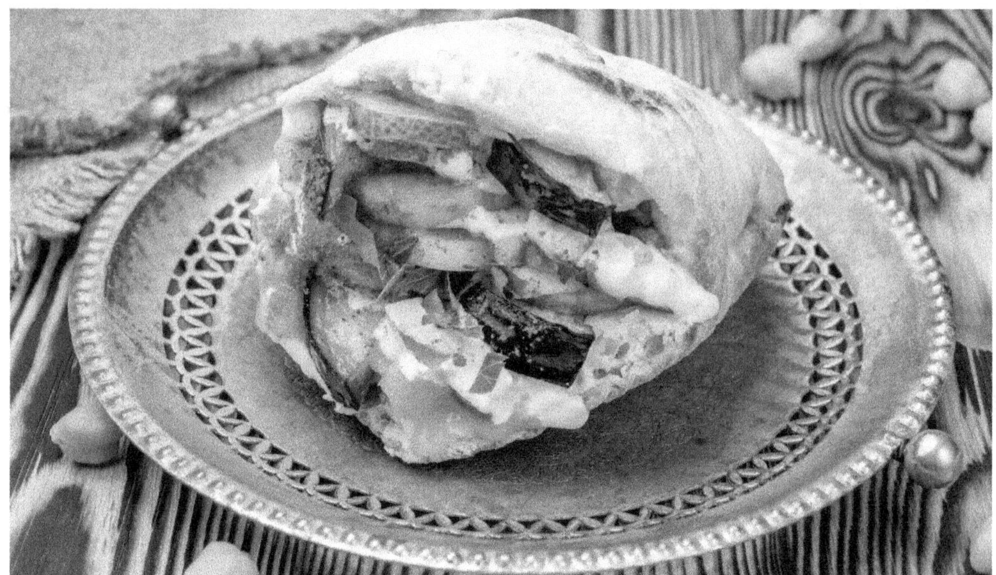

Preparation Time: 10 minutes

Cooking Time: 10 minutes

Servings: 4

Ingredients:

- 1/2 cup cooked white beans
- 2 medium potatoes, peeled, boiled, ½-inch thick sliced
- 1 medium eggplant, destemmed, ½-inch cubed
- 4 dill pickles, ¼-inch thick sliced
- ¼ teaspoon of sea salt
- 2 tablespoons olive oil
- 1/4 teaspoon harissa paste
- 1/2 cup hummus
- 1 tablespoon mayonnaise
- 4 pita bread pockets
- 1/2 cup tabbouleh salad

Directions:

1. Take a small frying pan, place it over medium-low heat, add oil and wait until it gets hot.

2. Season eggplant pieces with salt, add to the hot frying pan and cook for 8 minutes until softened, and when done, remove the pan from heat.

3. Take a small bowl, place white beans in it, add harissa paste and mayonnaise and then stir until combined.

4. Assemble the sandwich and for this, place pita bread on clean working space, smear generously with hummus, then cover half of each pita bread with potato slices and top with a dill pickle slices.

5. Spoon 2 tablespoons of white bean mixture on each dill pickle, top with 3 tablespoons of cooked eggplant pieces and 2 tablespoons of tabbouleh salad and then cover the filling with the other half of pita bread.

6. Serve straight away.

Nutrition:

386 Cal

13 g Fat

2 g Saturated Fat

56 g Carbohydrates

7 g Fiber

3 g Sugars

12 g Protein;

13. Tofu and Pesto Sandwich

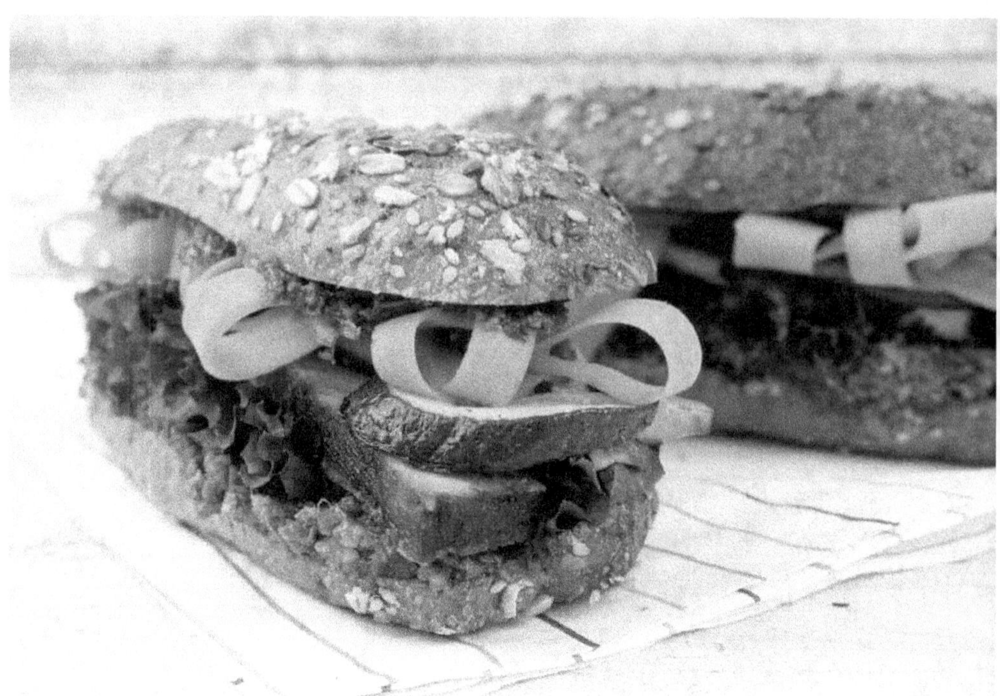

Preparation Time: 10 minutes

Cooking Time: 15 minutes

Servings: 4

Ingredients:

- 2 blocks of tofu, firm, pressed, drain
- 8 slices of tomato
- 8 leaves of lettuce
- 1 ½ teaspoon dried oregano
- ½ cup green pesto
- 2 tablespoons olive oil
- 8 slices of sandwich bread

Directions:

1. Cut tofu into thick slices, place them in a baking sheet, drizzle with oil and sprinkle with oregano, and bake the tofu pieces for 15 minutes until roasted.

2. Assemble the sandwich and for this, spread pesto on one side of each bread slice, then top four slices with lettuce, tomato slices, and roasted tofu and then cover with the other four slices.
3. Serve straight away.

Nutrition:

277 Cal

9.1 g Fat

1.5 g Saturated Fat

33.1 g Carbohydrates

3.6 g Fiber

12.7 g Sugars

16.1 g Protein;

14. Chickpea and Mayonnaise Salad Sandwich

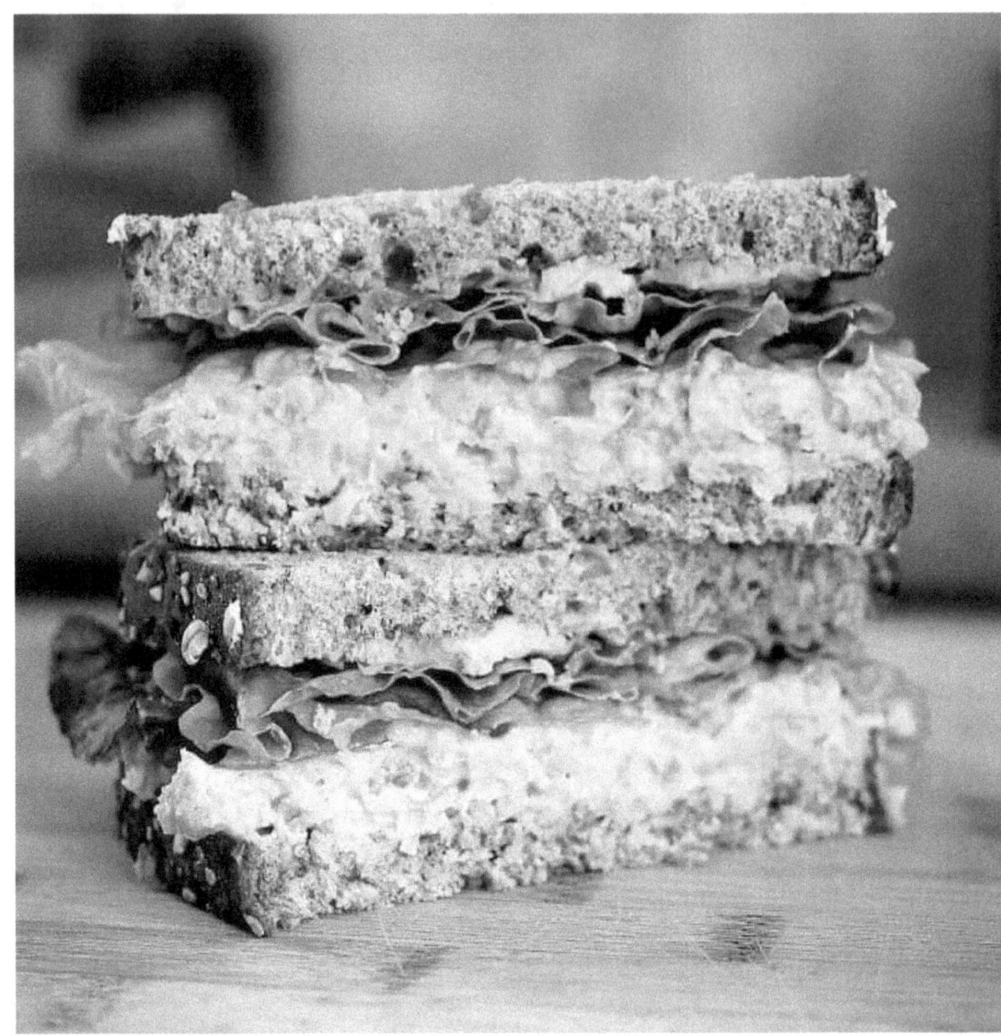

Preparation Time: 10 minutes

Cooking Time: 0 minutes

Servings: 4

Ingredients:

For the mayonnaise:

- 1/3 cup cashew nuts, soaked in boiling water for 10 minutes
- ½ teaspoon ground black pepper

- 1 teaspoon salt
- 6 teaspoons apple cider vinegar
- 2 teaspoon maple syrup
- 1/2 teaspoon Dijon mustard

For the chickpea salad:

- 1 small bunch of chives, chopped
- 1 ½ cup sweetcorn
- 3 cups cooked chickpeas

To serve:

- 4 sandwich bread
- 4 leaves of lettuce
- ½ cup chopped cherry tomatoes

Directions:

1. Prepare the mayonnaise and for this, place all of its ingredients in a food processor and then pulse for 2 minutes until smooth, scraping the sides of the container frequently.
2. Take a medium bowl, place chickpeas in it, and then mash by using a fork until broken.
3. Add chives and corn, stir until mixed, then add mayonnaise and stir until well combined.
4. Assemble the sandwich and for this, stuff sandwich bread with chickpea salad, top each sandwich with a lettuce leaf, and ¼ cup of chopped tomatoes and then serve.

Nutrition:

387 Cal

19 g Fat

5 g Saturated Fat

39.7 g Carbohydrates

7.2 g Fiber

4.6 g Sugars

10 g Protein;

15. Mushrooms Sandwich

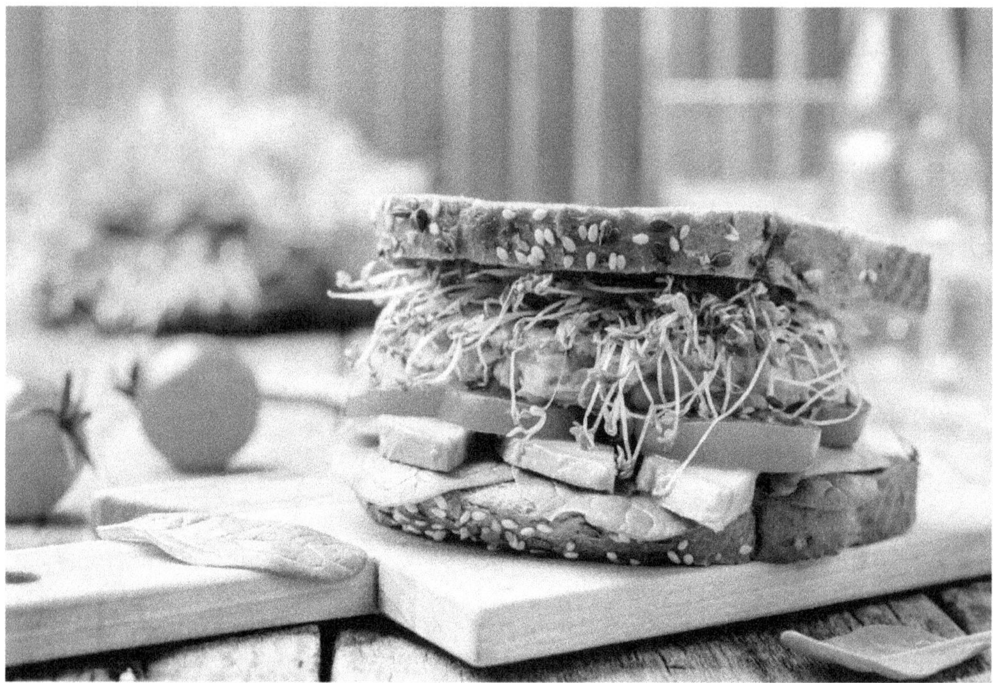

Preparation Time: 10 minutes

Cooking Time: 5 minutes

Servings: 4

Ingredients:

- 8 cherry tomatoes, halved
- 2 ounces of baby spinach
- 20 ounces of oyster mushrooms
- 2/3 teaspoon salt
- 1/3 teaspoon ground black pepper
- 2 tablespoons olive oil
- 4 tablespoons of barbecue sauce
- 8 slices of bread, toasted

Directions:

1. Take a griddle pan, place it over medium-high heat, grease it with oil and let it preheat.

2. Cut mushroom into thin strips, add to the hot griddle pan, drizzle with oil and cook for 5 minutes until done.
3. Transfer grilled mushrooms into a medium bowl, season with salt and black pepper, add barbecue sauce and toss until mixed.
4. Spread prepared mushroom mixture evenly on four bread slices, top with spinach and cherry tomatoes, then cover with the other four slices and serve.

Nutrition:

350 Cal

11 g Fat

3 g Saturated Fat

46 g Carbohydrates

9 g Fiber

7.2 g Sugars

12.1 g Protein;

16. Rainbow Taco Boats

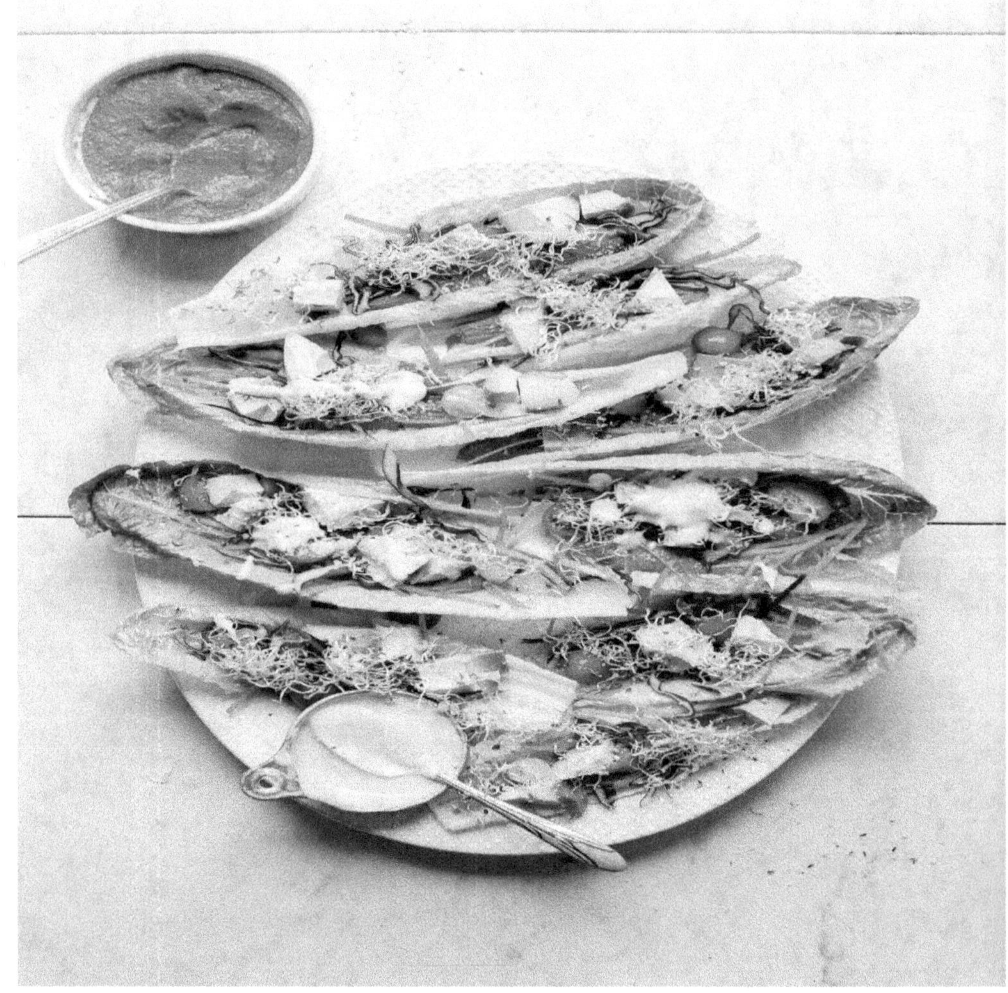

Preparation Time: 10 minutes

Cooking Time: 0 minutes

Servings: 4

Ingredients:

- 1 head romaine lettuce, destemmed

For the Filling:

- 1/2 cup alfalfa sprouts

- 1 medium avocado, peeled, pitted, cubed
- 1 cup shredded carrots
- 1 cup halved cherry tomatoes
- 3/4 cup sliced red cabbage
- 1/2 cup sprouted hummus dip
- 1 tablespoon hemp seeds

For the Sauce:

- 1 tablespoon maple syrup
- 1/3 cup tahini
- 1/8 teaspoon sea salt
- 2 tablespoons lemon juice
- 3 tablespoons water

Directions:

1. Prepare the sauce and for this, take a medium bowl, add all the ingredients in it and whisk until well combined.
2. Assemble the boats and for this, arrange lettuce leaves in twelve portions, top each with hummus, and the remaining ingredients for the filling.
3. Serve with prepared sauce.

Nutrition:

314 Cal

23.6 g Fat

4 g Saturated Fat

23.2 g Carbohydrates

9.3 g Fiber

6.2 g Sugars

8 g Protein;

Chapter 6.   Dinner Recipes

17. Dijon Maple Burgers

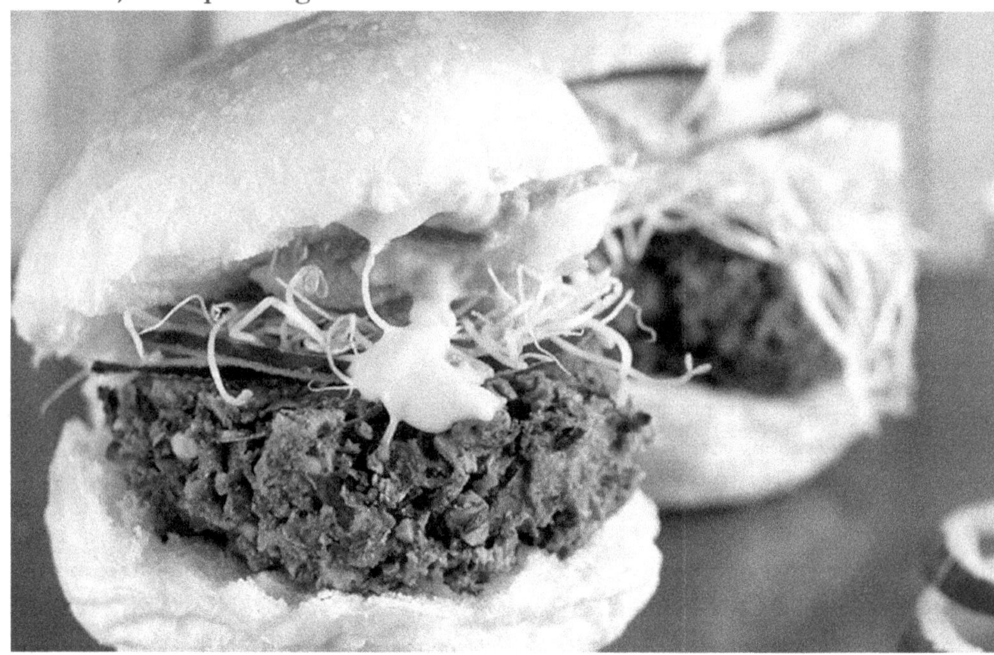

Preparation Time: 20 minutes

Cooking Time: 30 minutes

Servings: 12

Ingredients:

- 1 Red Bell Pepper
- 19 ounces Can Chickpeas, rinsed & drained
- 1 cup Almonds, ground
- 2 teaspoons Dijon Mustard
- 1 teaspoon Oregano
- ½ teaspoon Sage
- 1 cup Spinach, fresh
- 1 – ½ cups Rolled Oats
- 1 Clove Garlic, pressed
- ½ Lemon, juiced

- 2 teaspoons Maple Syrup, pure

Directions:

1. Get out a baking sheet. Line it with parchment paper.
2. Cut your red pepper in half and then take the seeds out. Place it on your baking sheet, and roast in the oven while you prepare your other ingredients.
3. Process your chickpeas, almonds, mustard, and maple syrup together in a food processor.
4. Add in your lemon juice, oregano, sage, garlic, and spinach, processing again. Make sure it's combined, but don't puree it.
5. Once your red bell pepper is softened, which should roughly take ten minutes, add this to the processor as well. Add in your oats, mixing well.
6. Form twelve patties, cooking in the oven for a half-hour. They should be browned.

Nutrition:

Calories: 96 kcal

Protein: 5.28 g

Fat: 2.42 g

Carbohydrates: 16.82 g

18. Hearty Black Lentil Curry

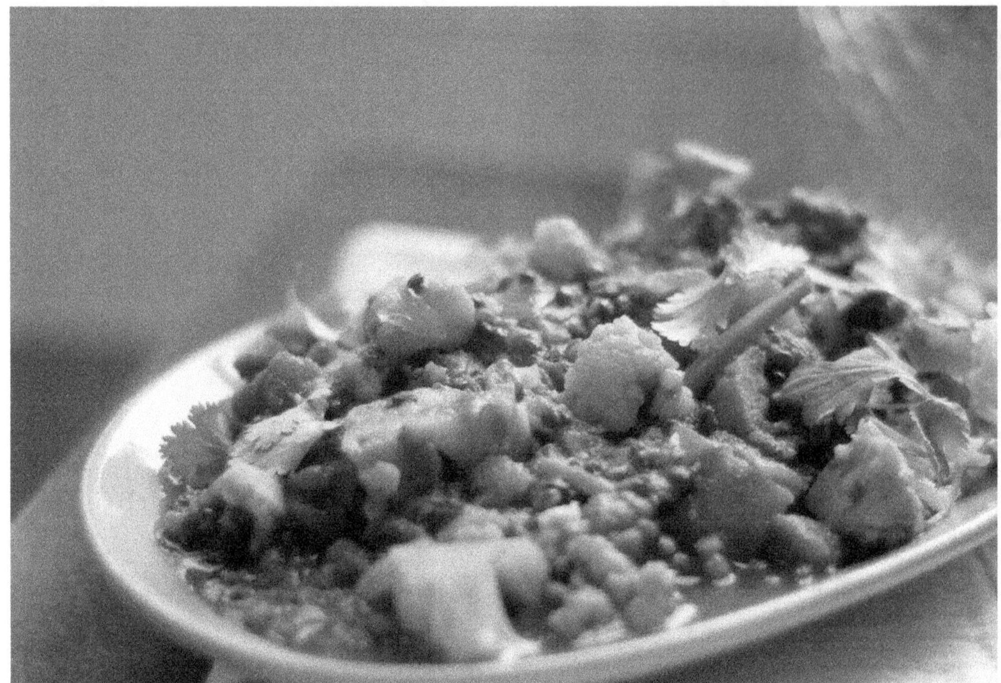

Preparation Time: 30 minutes

Cooking Time: 6 hours and 15 minutes

Servings: 4

Ingredients:

- 1 cup of black lentils, rinsed and soaked overnight
- 14 ounce of chopped tomatoes
- 2 large white onions, peeled and sliced
- 1 1/2 teaspoon of minced garlic
- 1 teaspoon of grated ginger
- 1 red chili
- 1 teaspoon of salt
- 1/4 teaspoon of red chili powder
- 1 teaspoon of paprika
- 1 teaspoon of ground turmeric
- 2 teaspoons of ground cumin
- 2 teaspoons of ground coriander

- 1/2 cup of chopped coriander
- 4-ounce of vegetarian butter
- 4 fluid of ounce water
- 2 fluid of ounce vegetarian double cream

Directions:

1. Place a large pan over moderate heat, add butter and let heat until melt.
2. Add the onion and garlic and ginger and cook for 10 to 15 minutes or until onions are caramelized.
3. Then stir in salt, red chili powder, paprika, turmeric, cumin, ground coriander, and water.
4. Transfer this mixture to a 6-quarts slow cooker and add tomatoes and red chili.
5. Drain lentils, add to slow cooker, and stir until just mix.
6. Plugin slow cooker; adjust cooking time to 6 hours and let cook on low heat setting.
7. When the lentils are done, stir in cream and adjust the seasoning.
8. Serve with boiled rice or whole wheat bread.

Nutrition:

Calories: 299 kcal

Protein: 5.59 g

Fat: 27.92 g

Carbohydrates: 9.83 g

19. Spicy Black-Eyed Peas

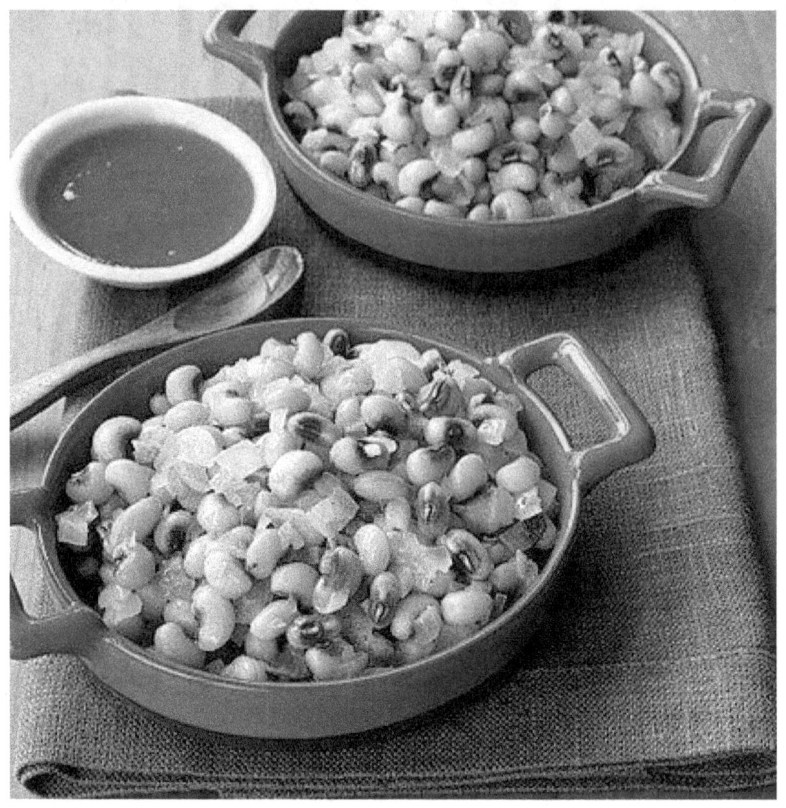

Preparation Time: 12 minutes

Cooking Time: 8 hours and 8 minutes

Servings: 8

Ingredients:

- 32-ounce black-eyed peas, uncooked
- 1 cup of chopped orange bell pepper
- 1 cup of chopped celery
- 8-ounce of chipotle peppers, chopped
- 1 cup of chopped carrot
- 1 cup of chopped white onion
- 1 teaspoon of minced garlic
- 3/4 teaspoon of salt
- 1/2 teaspoon of ground black pepper
- 2 teaspoons of liquid smoke flavoring
- 2 teaspoons of ground cumin
- 1 tablespoon of adobo sauce

- 2 tablespoons of olive oil
- 1 tablespoon of apple cider vinegar
- 4 cups of vegetable broth

Directions:

1. Place a medium-sized non-stick skillet pan over an average temperature of heat; add the bell peppers, carrot, onion, garlic, oil, and vinegar.
2. Stir until it mixes properly and let it cook for 5 to 8 minutes or until it gets translucent.
3. Transfer this mixture to a 6-quarts slow cooker and add the peas, chipotle pepper, adobo sauce, and the vegetable broth.
4. Stir until mixed properly and cover the top.
5. Connect the slow cooker, regulate the cooking time to 8 hours, and let it cook on the low heat setting or until peas are soft.
6. Serve right away.

Nutrition:

Calories: 1071 kcal

Protein: 5.3 g

Fat: 113.65 g

Carbohydrates: 18.51 g

20. Creamy Artichoke Soup

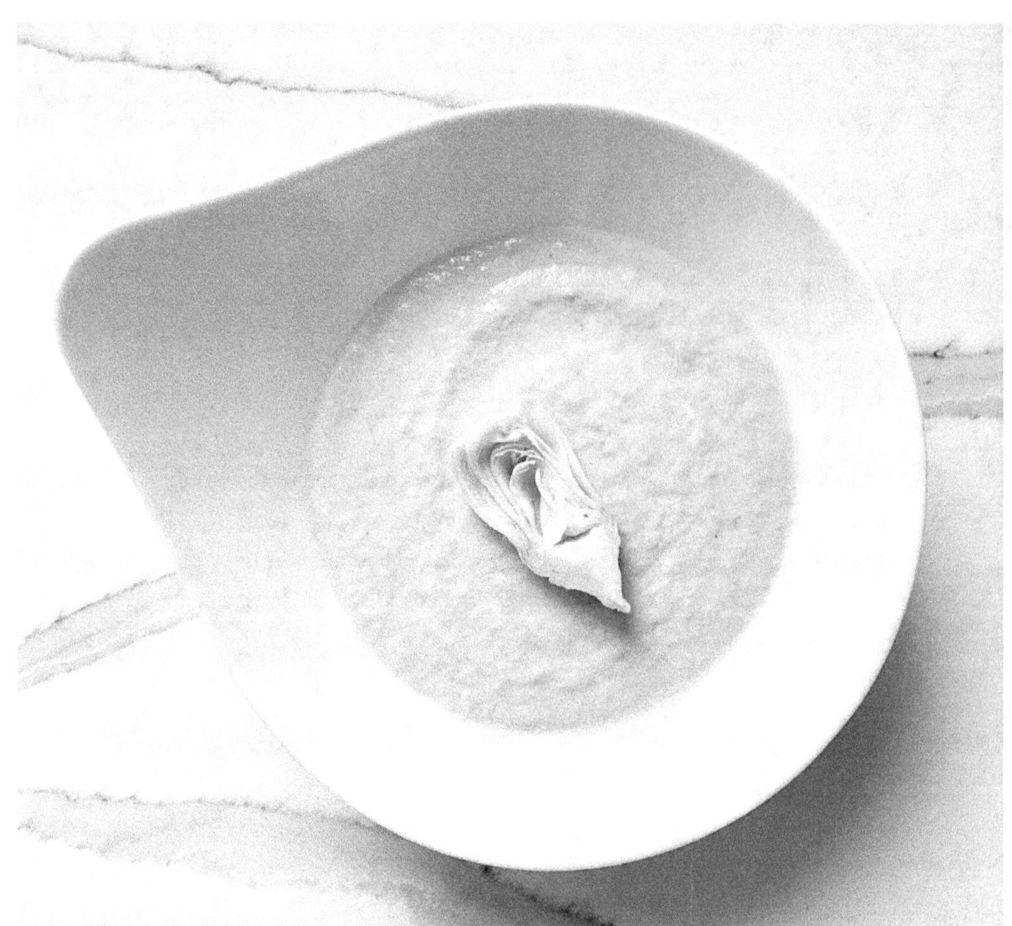

Preparation Time: 5 minutes

Cooking Time: 40 minutes

Servings: 4

Ingredients:

- 1 can artichoke hearts, drained
- 3 cups vegetable broth
- 2 tbsp. lemon juice
- 1 small onion, finely cut
- 2 cloves garlic, crushed
- 3 tbsp. olive oil
- 2 tbsp. flour

- ½ cup vegan cream

Directions:

1. Gently sauté the onion and garlic in some olive oil. Add the flour, whisking constantly, and then add the hot vegetable broth slowly, while still whisking. Cook for about 5 minutes.
2. Blend the artichoke, lemon juice, salt, and pepper until smooth. Add the puree to the broth mix, stir well, and then stir in the cream. Cook until heated through. Garnish with a swirl of vegan cream or a sliver of artichoke.

Nutrition:

Calories: 1622 kcal

Protein: 4.45 g

Fat: 181.08 g

Carbohydrates: 10.99 g

21. Tomato Artichoke Soup

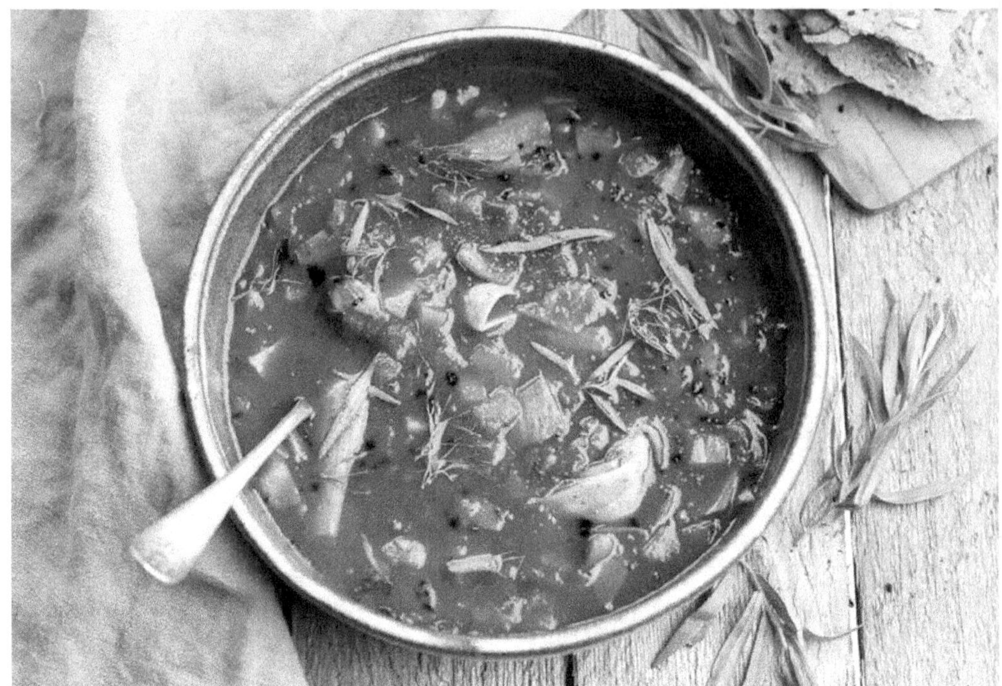

Preparation Time: 5 minutes

Cooking Time: 6 hours

Servings: 4

Ingredients:

- 1 can artichoke hearts, drained
- 1 can diced tomatoes, undrained
- 3 cups vegetable broth
- 1 small onion, chopped
- 2 cloves garlic, crushed
- 1 tbsp. pesto
- Black pepper, to taste

Directions:

1. Combine all ingredients in the slow cooker.
2. Cook on low for 10 hours or on high for 4-5 hours.

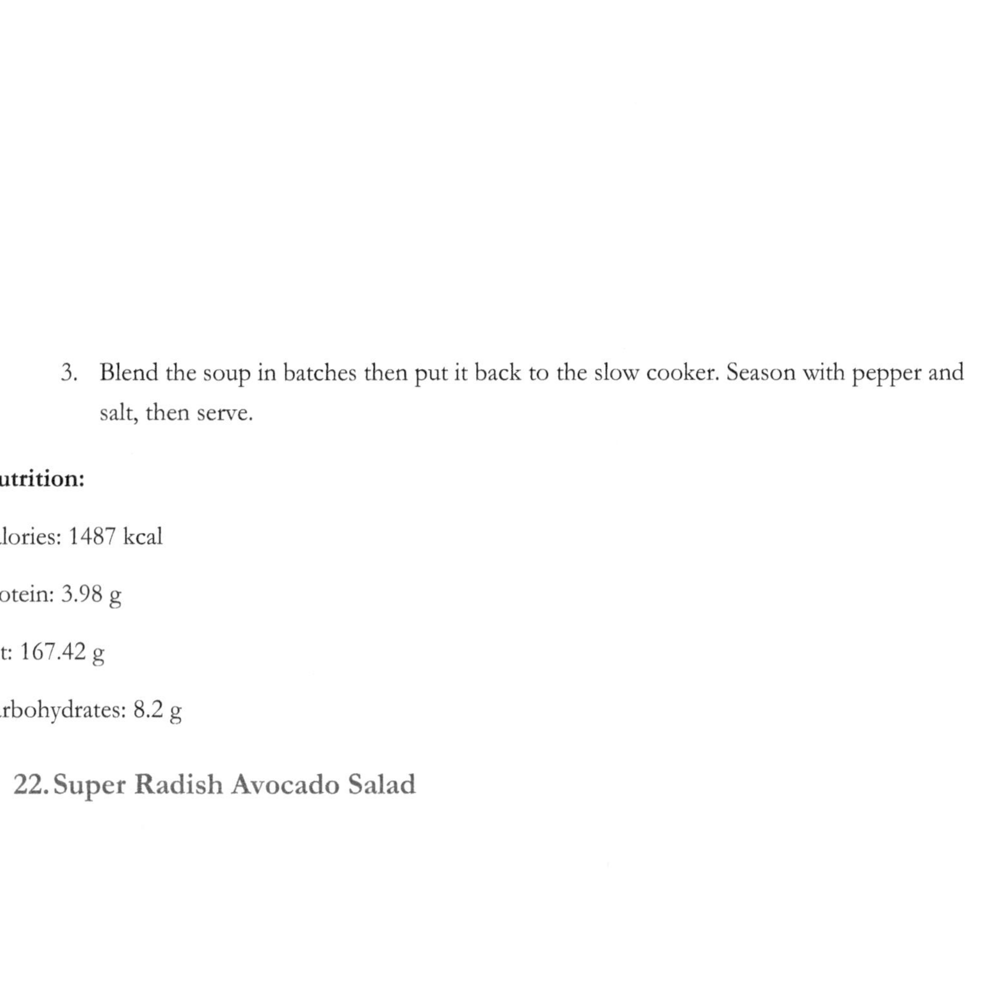

3. Blend the soup in batches then put it back to the slow cooker. Season with pepper and salt, then serve.

Nutrition:

Calories: 1487 kcal

Protein: 3.98 g

Fat: 167.42 g

Carbohydrates: 8.2 g

22. Super Radish Avocado Salad

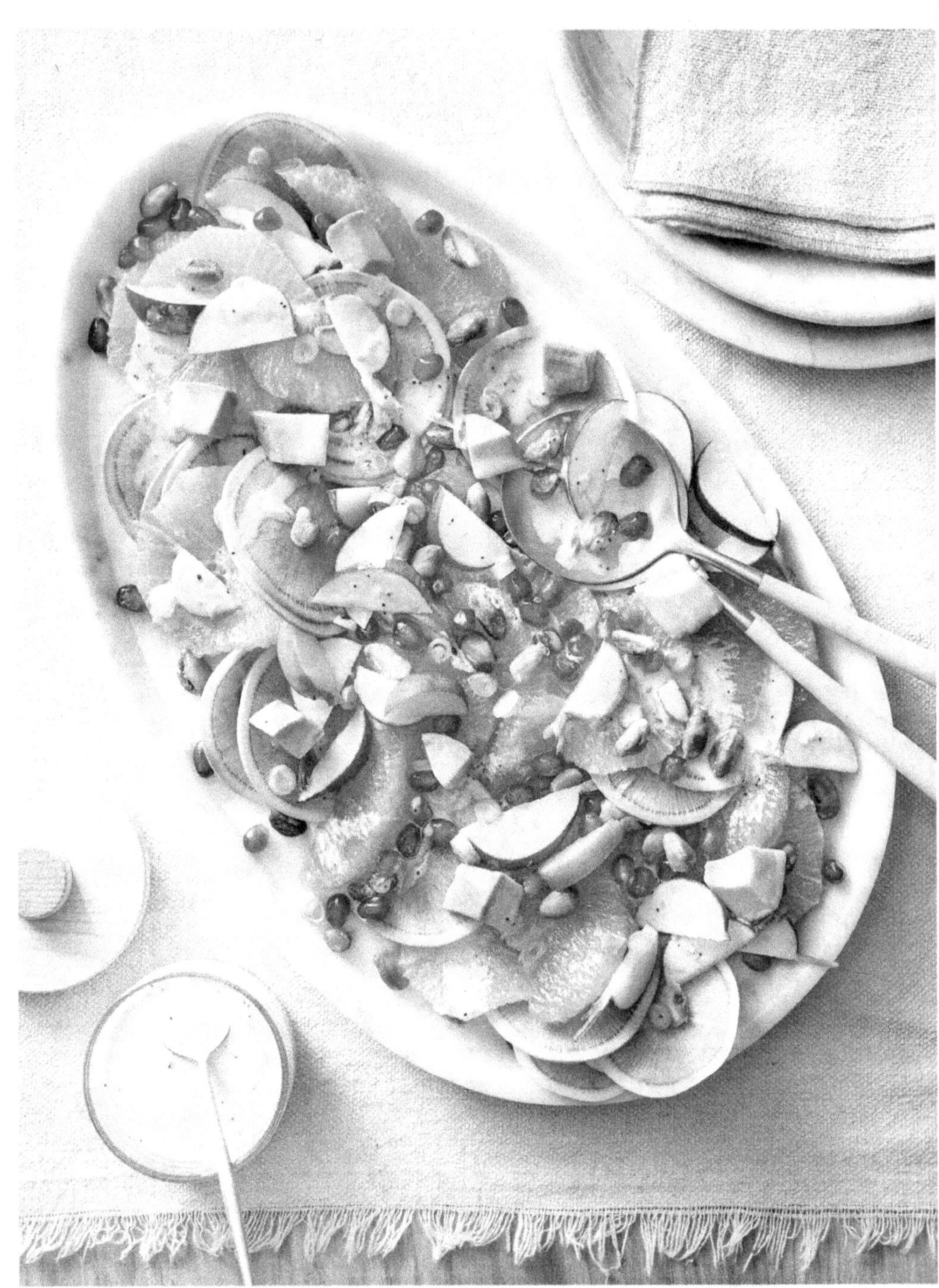

Preparation Time: 10 minutes

Cooking Time: 25 minutes

Servings: 2

Ingredients:

- 6 shredded carrots
- 6 ounces diced radishes
- 1 diced avocado
- 1/3 cup ponzu

Directions:

1. Place all together the ingredients in a serving bowl and toss. Enjoy!

Nutrition:

Calories: 292

kcal Protein: 7.42 g

Fat: 18.29 g

Carbohydrates: 29.59 g

23. Beauty School Ginger Cucumbers

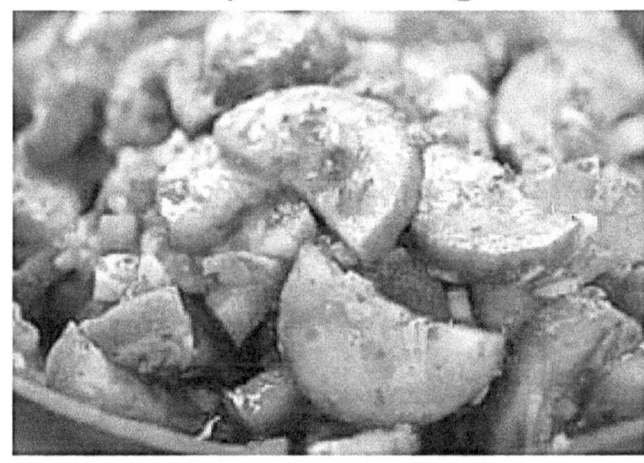

Preparation Time: 10 minutes

Cooking Time: 45 minutes

Servings: 14

Ingredients:

- 1 sliced cucumber
- 3 tsp. rice wine vinegar
- 1 ½ tbsp. sugar
- 1 tsp. minced ginger

Directions:

1. Place all together the ingredients in a mixing bowl, and toss the ingredients well. Enjoy!

Nutrition:

Calories: 10 kcal

Protein: 0.46 g

Fat: 0.43 g

Carbohydrates: 0.89 g

Chapter 7.   Snacks Recipes

24. Mango & Papaya After-Chop

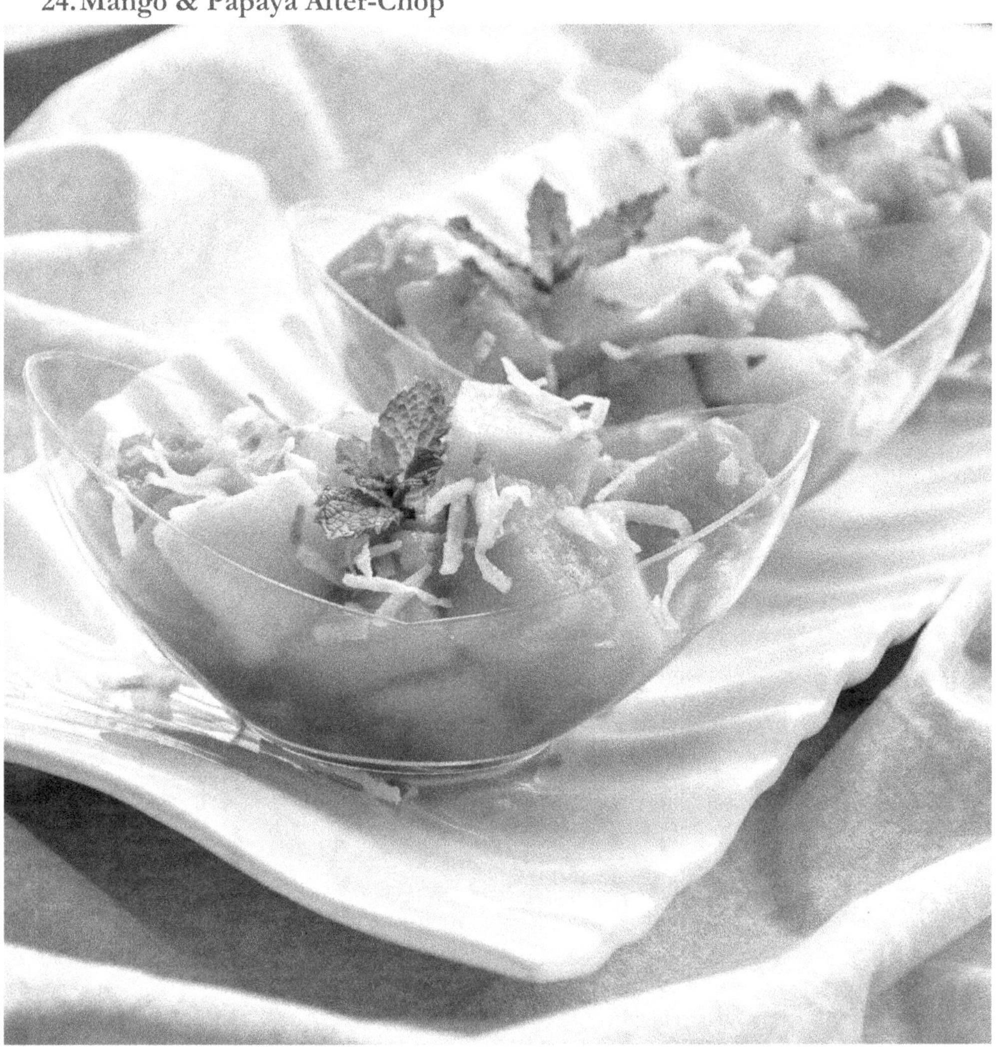

Preparation time: 25 minutes

Cooking time: 0 minutes

Servings: 4

Ingredients:

- 1/4 of papaya, chopped

- 1 mango, chopped
- 1 Tablespoon coconut milk
- 1/2 teaspoon maple syrup
- 1 Tablespoon peanuts, chopped

Directions:

1. Cut open the papaya. Scoop out the seeds, chop.
2. Peel the mango. Slice the fruit from the pit, chop.
3. Put the fruit in a bowl. Add remaining ingredients. Stir to coat.

Nutrition:

Calories 100,

Fats 1 g,

Carbohydrates 25 g,

Proteins 1 g

25. Sautéed Bosc Pears with Walnuts

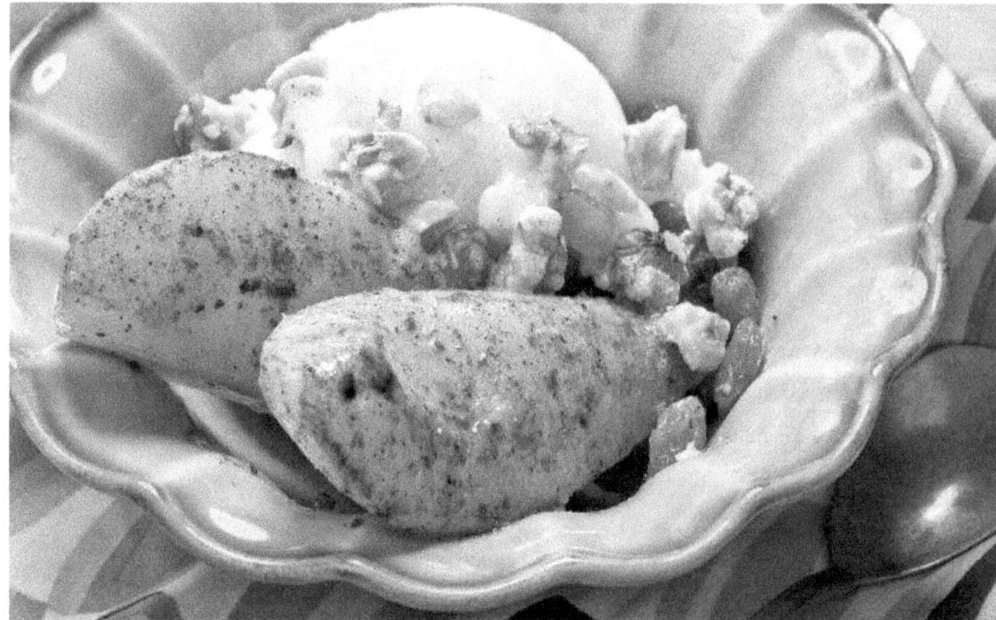

Preparation time: 15 minutes

Cooking time: 16 minutes

Servings: 6

Ingredients:

- 2 Tablespoon salted butter
- 1/4 teaspoon cinnamon
- 1/4 teaspoon nutmeg, ground
- 6 Bosc pears, peeled, quartered
- 1 Tablespoon lemon juice
- 1/2 cup walnuts, chopped, toasted

Directions:

1. Melt butter in a skillet, add spices and cook for 30 seconds.
2. Add pears and cook for 15 minutes. Stir in lemon juice.
3. Serve topped with walnuts.

Nutrition:

Calories 220,

Fats 10 g,

Carbohydrates 31 g,

Proteins 2 g

26. Brown Rice Pudding

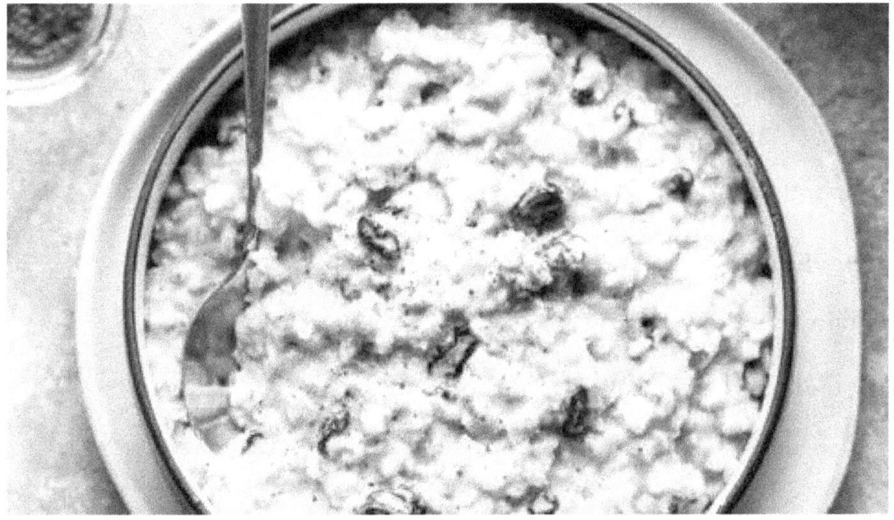

Preparation time: 5 minutes

Cooking time: 1 hour

Servings: 6

Ingredients:

- 2 cups brown rice, cooked
- 3 cups light coconut milk
- 3 eggs
- 1 cup brown sugar
- 1 teaspoon vanilla
- 1/2 teaspoon salt
- 1/2 teaspoon cinnamon
- 1/4 teaspoon nutmeg

Directions:

1. Blend all ingredients well. Put mixture in a 2-quart casserole dish.
2. Bake at 300 degree F for 90 minutes.
3. Serve.

Nutrition:

Calories 330,

Fats 10 g,

Carbohydrates 52 g,

Proteins 5 g

27. Date Porcupines

Preparation time: 20 minutes

Cooking time: 15 minutes

Servings: 18

Ingredients:

- 2 eggs
- 1 Tablespoon extra-virgin olive oil

- 1 teaspoon vanilla
- 1 cup Medjool dates, pitted, chopped
- 1 cup walnuts, chopped
- 3/4 cup flour
- 1 cup coconut, shredded
- 1/2 teaspoon salt

Directions:

1. Preheat oven to 350 degree F.
2. Beat the eggs, adding the oil and vanilla. Fold in the dates and walnuts. Form the mix into small balls and roll in coconut. Bake for 15 minutes.
3. Serve cold.

Nutrition:

Calories 114,

Fats 1 g,

Carbohydrates 8 g,

Proteins 1 g

28. Raspberry Chia Pudding Shots

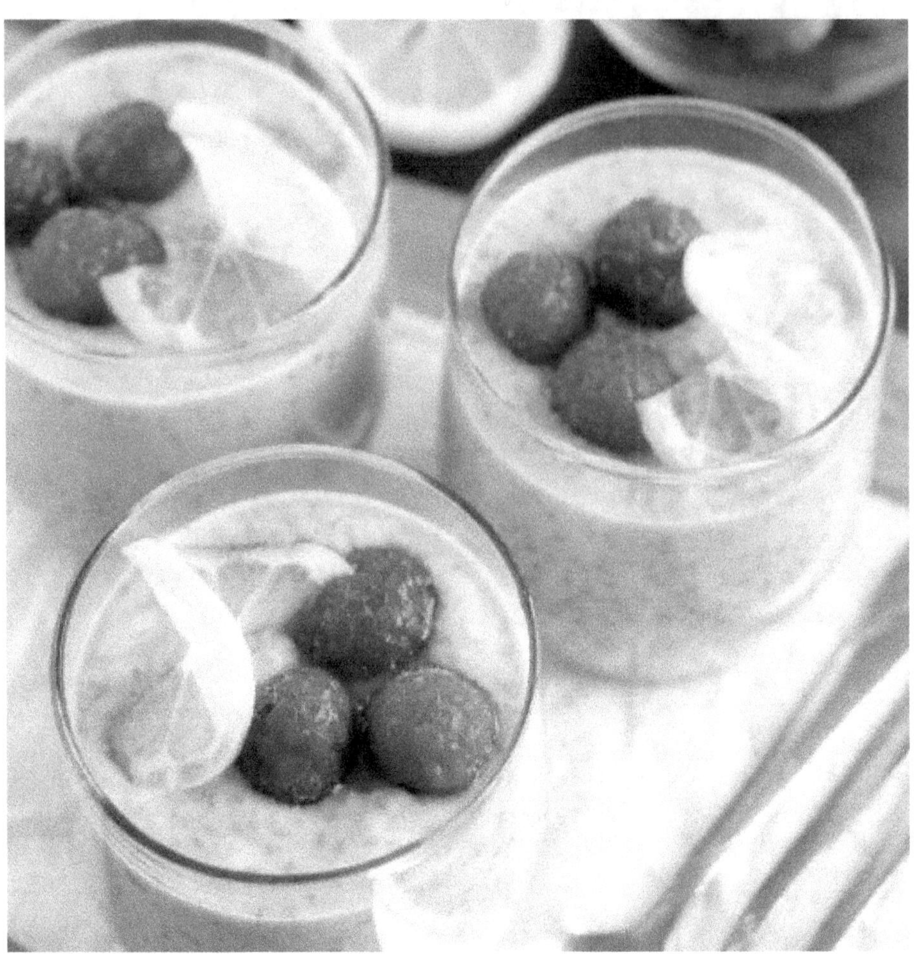

Preparation time: 1 hour

Cooking time: 15 minutes

Servings: 12

Ingredients:

- 1/4 cup chia seeds
- 1/2 cup raspberries
- 1/2 cup coconut milk
- 1/4 cup almond milk
- 1 Tablespoon cacao powder
- 1 Tablespoon stevia

Directions:

1. Combine all ingredients except raspberries in a jar.

2. Let sit for 2-3 minutes and transfer to shot glasses.

3. Refrigerate 1 hour, or overnight to serve as breakfast.

4. Serve with fresh raspberries.

Nutrition:

Calories 240,

Fats 19 g,

Carbohydrates 5 g,

Proteins 5 g

29. Banana Muffins

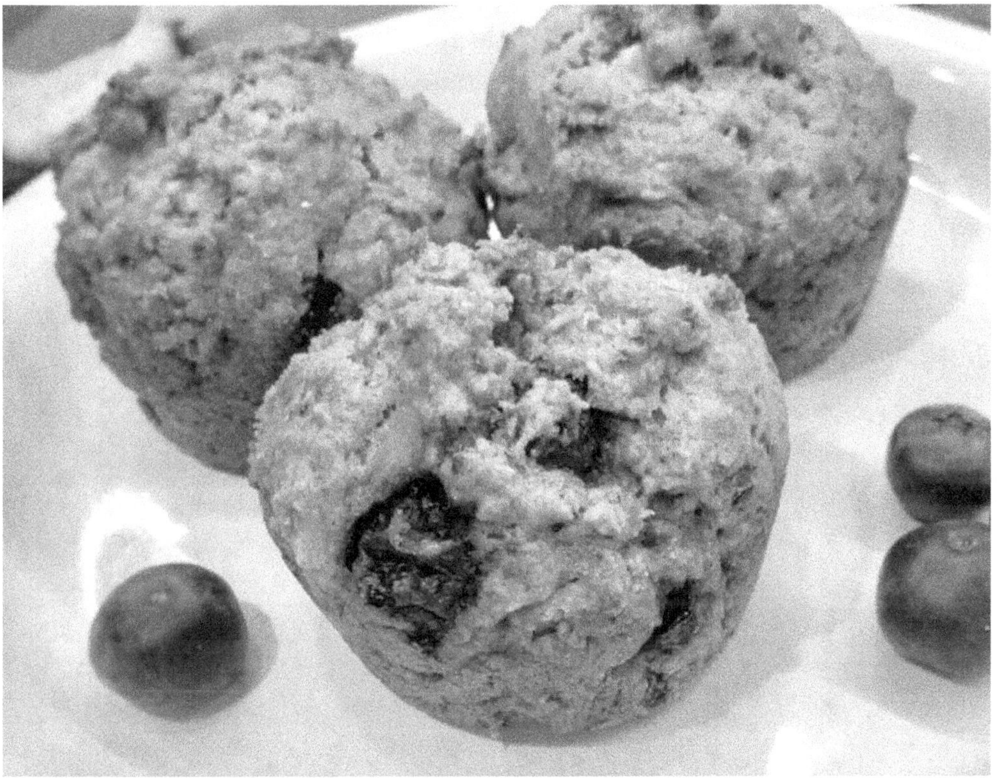

Preparation time: 15 minutes

Cooking time: 15 minutes

Servings: 18

Ingredients:

- 3 bananas
- 2 eggs
- 2 cups whole wheat pastry flour
- 1/3 cup sugar
- 1 teaspoon salt
- 1 teaspoon baking soda
- 1/2 cup walnuts, chopped

Directions:

1. Preheat oven to 350 degree F.
2. Grease 10 cups of a muffin tin.
3. Mix bananas and eggs together. Add sifted dry ingredients.
4. Add nuts. Mix well.
5. Spoon into muffin tins. Bake for 20 minutes.

Nutrition:

Calories 108,

Fats 1 g,

Carbohydrates 8 g,

Proteins 1 g

Chapter 8.   Dips and sauces Recipes

30. Avocado Bean Dip

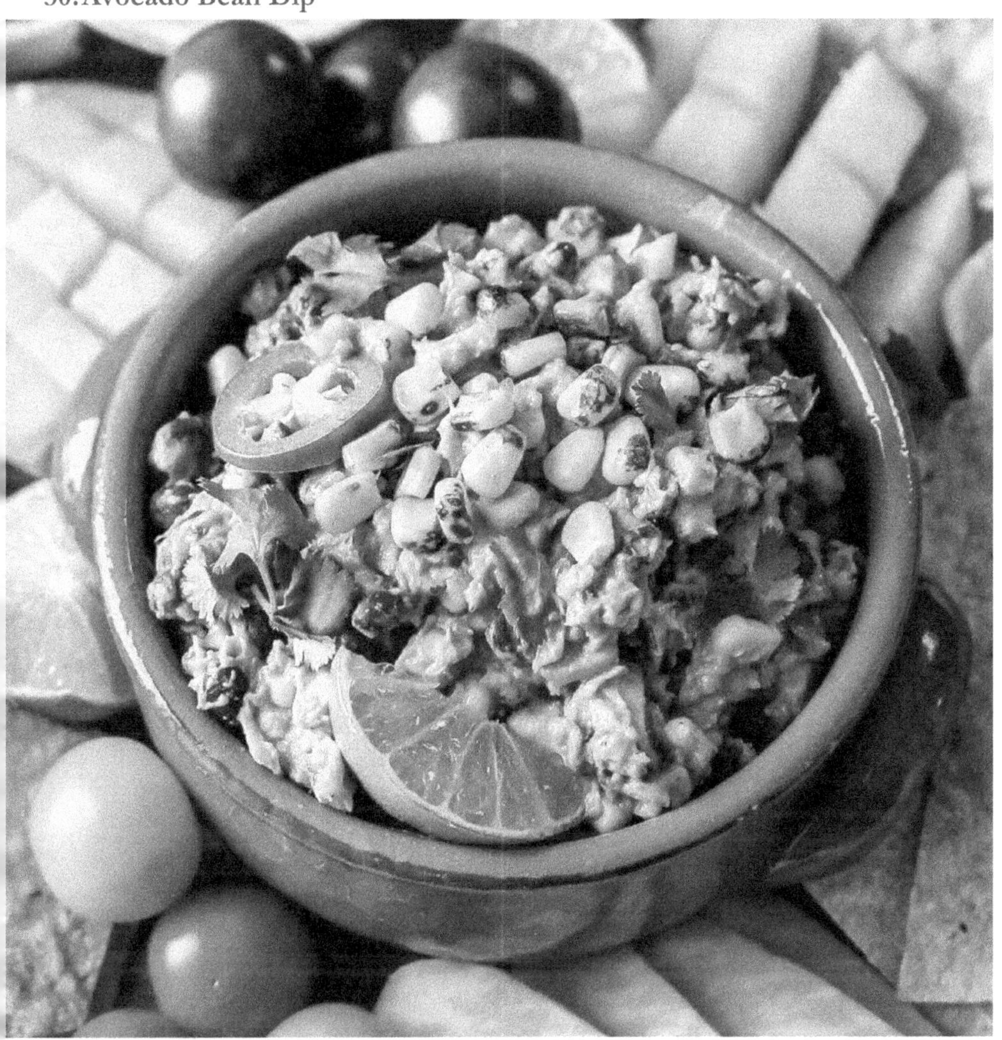

Preparation Time: 15 minutes

Cooking Time: 15 minutes

Servings: 2

Ingredients:

- 1 medium ripe avocado, peeled and cubed

- 1/2 cup fresh cilantro leaves
- 3 tablespoon lime juice
- 1/2 teaspoon onion powder
- 1/2 teaspoon garlic powder
- 1/2 teaspoon chipotle hot pepper sauce
- 1/4 teaspoon salt
- 1/4 teaspoon ground cumin
- Baked tortilla chips

Directions:

1. Mix all the fixings in a food processor, then cover and blend until smooth. Serve along with chips.

Nutrition:

Calories 85

Fat 4

Carbs 13

Protein 6

31. Creamy Cucumber Yogurt Dip

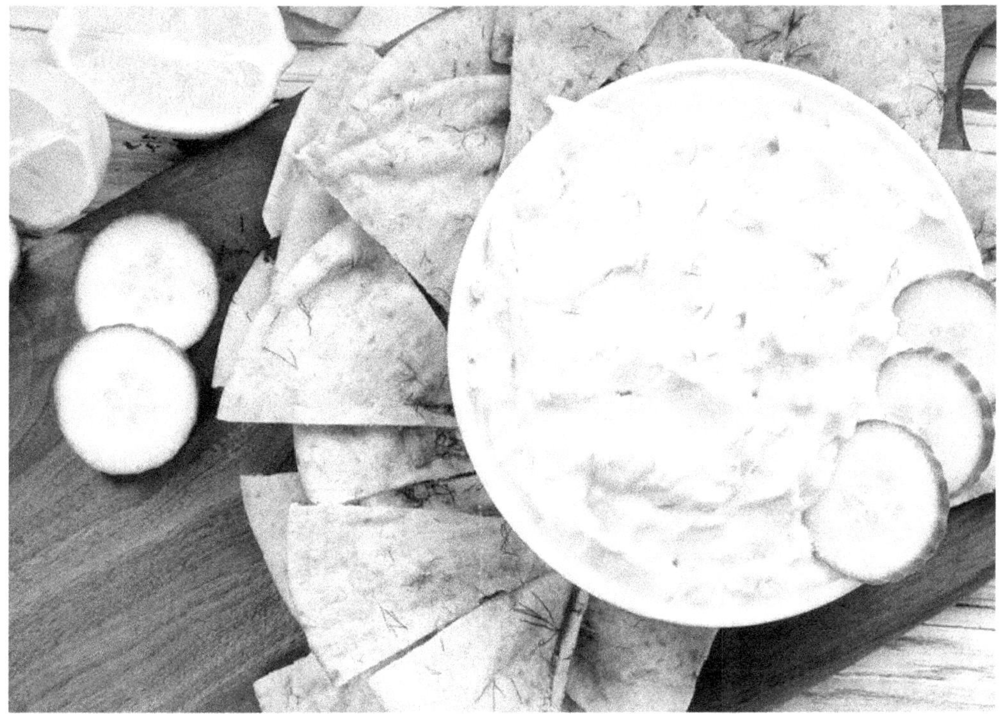

Preparation Time: 15 minutes

Cooking Time: 15 minutes

Servings: 4

Ingredients:

- 1 cup (8 oz.) reduced-Fat plain yogurt
- 4 oz. reduced-Fat cream cheese
- 1/2 cup chopped seeded peeled cucumber
- 1-1/2 teaspoon. finely chopped onion
- 1-1/2 teaspoon. snipped fresh dill
- 1 teaspoon lemon juice
- 1 teaspoon grated lemon peel
- 1 garlic clove, minced
- 1/4 teaspoon salt
- 1/4 teaspoon pepper
- Assorted fresh vegetables

Directions:

1. Mix the cream cheese and yogurt in a small bowl. Stir in pepper, salt, garlic, peel, lemon juice, dill, onion, and cucumber. Put on the cover and let it chill in the fridge. Serve it with the veggies.

Nutrition:

Calories 55

Fat 4

Carbs 12

Protein 6

32. Garlic White Bean Dip

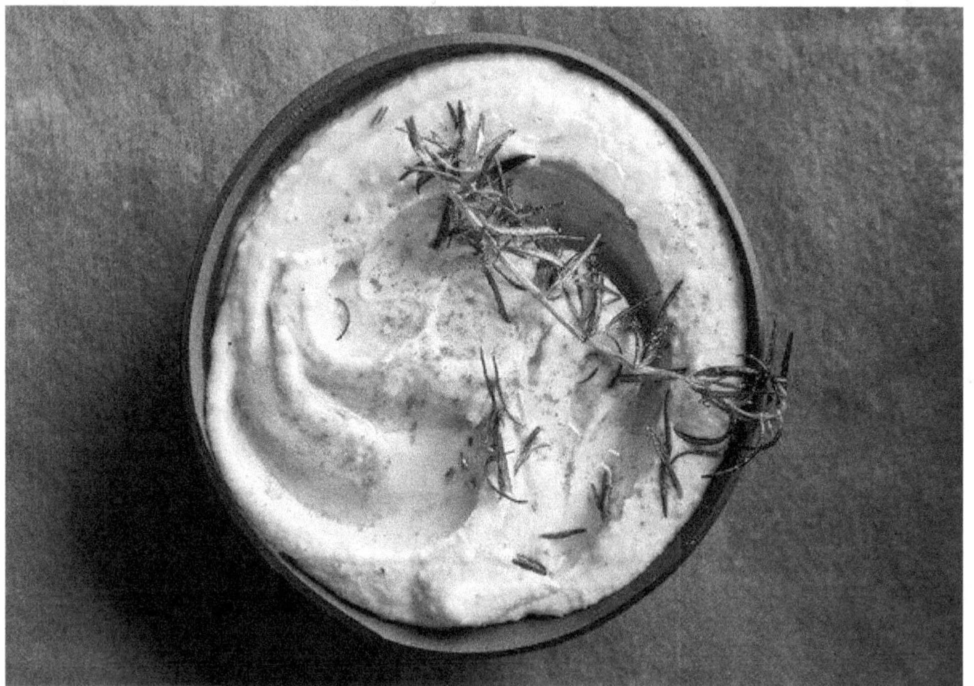

Preparation Time: 15 minutes

Cooking Time: 15 minutes

Servings: 2

Ingredients:

- 1/4 cup soft bread crumbs
- 2 tablespoon dry white wine or water
- 2 tablespoon olive oil
- 2 tablespoon lemon juice
- 4-1/2 teaspoon. minced fresh parsley
- 3 garlic cloves, peeled and halved
- 1/2 teaspoon salt
- 1/4 teaspoon dill weed
- 1/8 teaspoon cayenne pepper
- Assorted fresh vegetables

Directions:

1. Mix wine and bread crumbs in a small bowl. Mix cayenne, dill, salt, garlic, parsley, beans, lemon juice, and oil in a food processor, then cover and blend until smooth.
2. Put in bread crumb mixture and process until well combined. Serve together with vegetables.

Nutrition:

Calories 105

Fat 5

Carbs 12

Protein 6

33. Satay Sauce

Preparation Time: 5 minutes

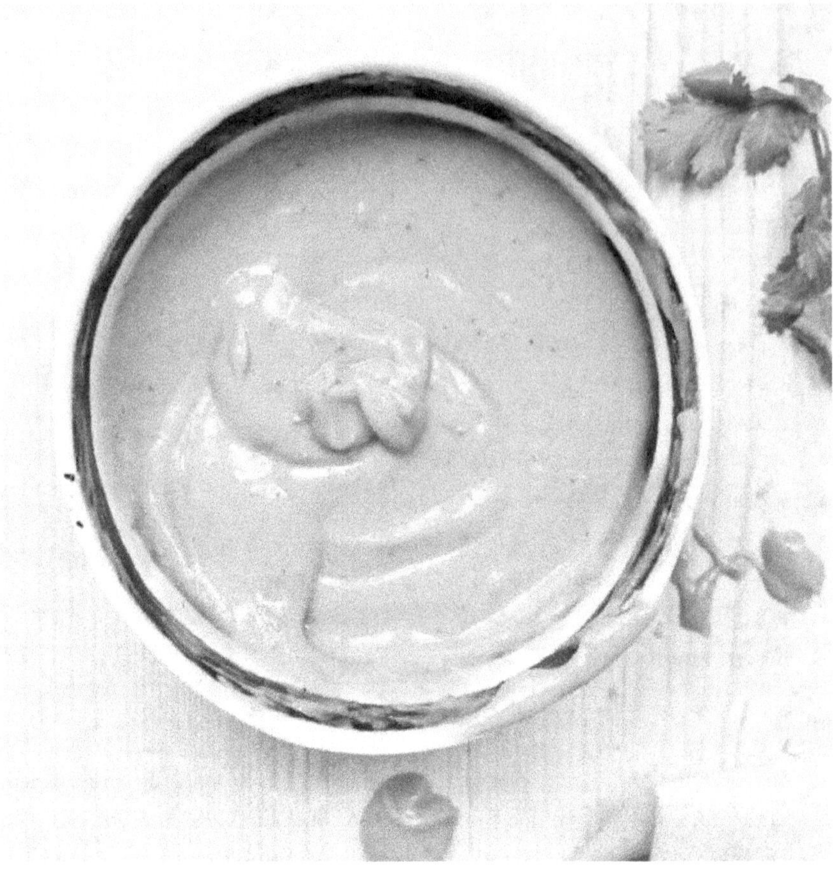

Cooking Time: 8 minutes

Servings: 2

Ingredients:

- ½ yellow onion, diced
- 3 garlic cloves, minced
- 1 fresh red chile, thinly sliced (optional)
- ¼ cup smooth peanut butter
- 2 tablespoons coconut aminos
- 1 (13.5-ounce / 383-g) can unsweetened coconut milk
- ¼ teaspoon freshly ground black pepper
- ¼ teaspoon salt (optional)

Directions:

1. Heat a skillet over heat until hot.

2. Add the onion, garlic cloves, chile (if desired), and ginger to the skillet, and sauté for 2 minutes.
3. Pour in the peanut butter and coconut aminos and stir well. Add the coconut milk, black pepper, and salt (if desired) and continue whisking, or until the sauce is just beginning to bubble and thicken.
4. Remove the sauce from the heat to a bowl. Taste and adjust the seasoning if necessary.

Nutrition:

Calories: 322

Fat: 28.8g

Carbs: 9.4g

Protein: 6.3g

Fiber: 1.8g

34. Tamari Vinegar Sauce

Preparation Time: 10 minutes

Cooking Time: 0 minutes

Servings: 1

Ingredients:

- ¼ cup tamari
- ½ cup nutritional yeast
- 2 tablespoons balsamic vinegar
- 2 tablespoons apple cider vinegar
- 2 tablespoons Worcestershire sauce
- 2 teaspoons Dijon mustard
- 1 tablespoon plus 1 teaspoon maple syrup
- ½ teaspoon ground turmeric
- ¼ teaspoon black pepper

Directions:

1. Place all the ingredients in an airtight container, and whisk until everything is well incorporated. Store in the refrigerator for up to 3 weeks.

Nutrition:

Calories: 216

Fat: 9.9g

Carbs: 18.0g

Protein: 13.7g

Fiber: 7.7g

Chapter 9.   Soup and Stew

35. Moroccan Vegetable Stew

Preparation Time: 5 minutes

Cooking Time: 35 minutes

Servings: 4

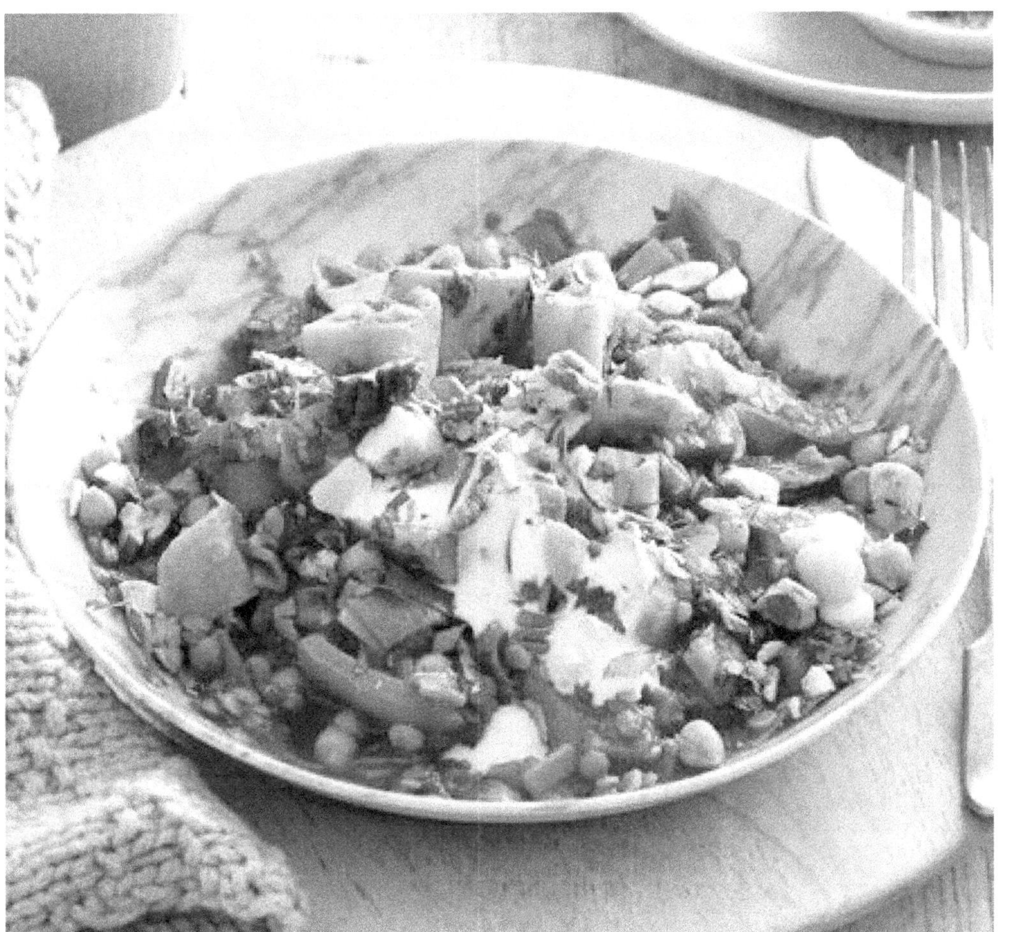

Ingredients:

- 1 tablespoon olive oil
- 2 medium yellow onions, chopped
- 2 medium carrots

- 1/2 teaspoon ground cumin
- 1/2 teaspoon ground cinnamon or allspice
- 1/2 teaspoon ground ginger
- 1/2 teaspoon sweet or smoked paprika
- 1/2 teaspoon saffron or turmeric
- 1 (14.5-ounce) can diced tomatoes, undrained
- 8 ounces green beans
- 2 cups peeled, seeded, and diced winter squash
- 1 large russet or other baking potato, peeled and cut into 1/2-inch dice
- 11/2 cups vegetable broth
- 11/2 cups cooked can chickpeas, drained and rinsed
- ¾ cup frozen peas
- 1/2 cup pitted dried plums (prunes)
- 1 teaspoon lemon zest
- Salt and freshly ground black pepper
- 1/2 cup pitted green olives
- 1 tablespoon minced fresh cilantro or parsley, for garnish
- 1/2 cup toasted slivered almonds, for garnish

Directions:

1. In a pan, heat the oil over heat. Add the onions and carrots, cover, and cook for 5 minutes. Stir in the cumin, cinnamon, ginger, paprika, and saffron. Cook, uncovered, stirring, for 30 seconds.
2. Add the tomatoes, green beans, squash, potato, and broth and bring to a boil.
3. Add the chickpeas, peas, dried plums, and lemon zest. Season with salt and pepper to taste. Stir in the olives and simmer, uncovered, until the flavors are blended, about 10 minutes. Sprinkle with cilantro and almonds and serve immediately.

Nutrition:

Calories: 71 Calories

Fat: 2.8g

Carbs: 9.8g

Protein: 3.7g

36. Basic Recipe for Vegetable Broth

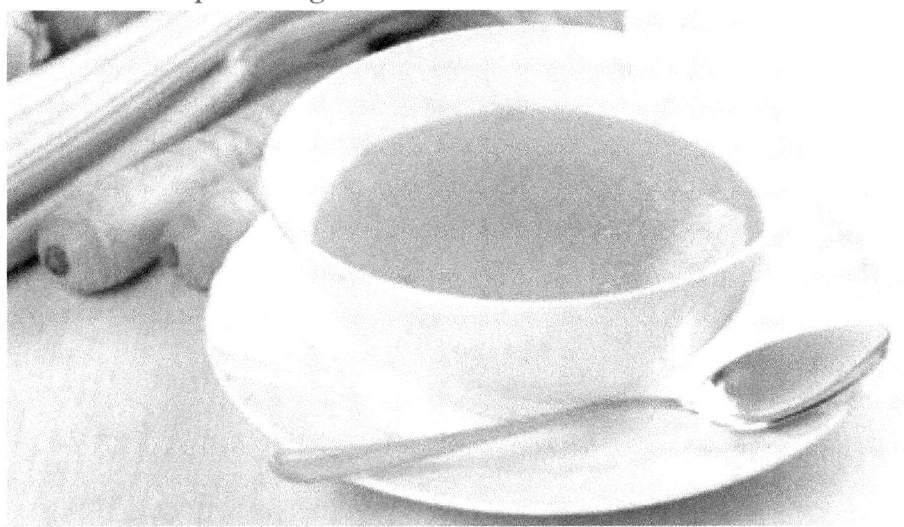

Preparation Time: 10 Minutes

Cooking Time: 60 Minutes

Servings: Makes 2 Quarts

Ingredients:

- 8 cups Water
- 1 Onion, chopped
- 4 Garlic cloves, crushed
- 2 Celery Stalks, chopped
- Pinch of Salt
- 1 Carrot, chopped
- Dash of Pepper
- 1 Potato, medium & chopped
- 1 tbsp. Soy Sauce
- 3 Bay Leaves

Directions:

1. To make the vegetable broth, you need to place all of the ingredients in a deep saucepan.
2. Heat the pan over a medium-high heat. Bring the vegetable mixture to a boil.

3. Once it starts steaming, lower the heat to medium-low and allow it to simmer for at least an hour or so. Cover it with a lid.

4. When the time is up, pass it through a filter and strain the vegetables, garlic, and bay leaves.

5. Allow the stock to cool completely and store in an air-tight container.

Nutrition:

Calories: 44 Calories

Fat: 0.6g

Carbs: 9.7g

Protein: 0.9g

37. Cabbage & Beet Stew

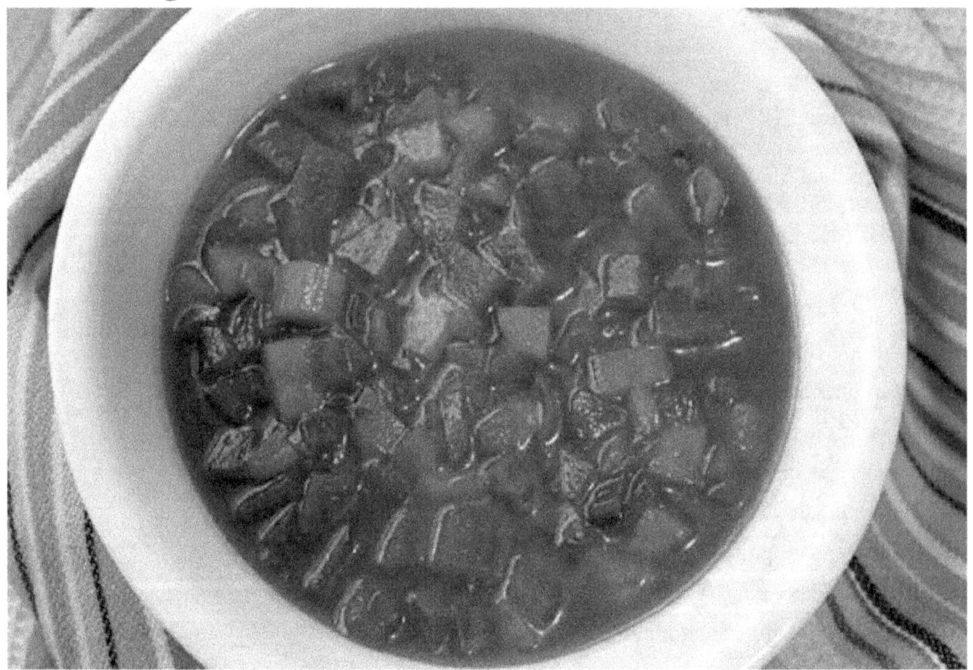

Preparation Time: 20 minutes

Cooking Time: 10 minutes

Servings: 4

Ingredients:

- 2 Tablespoons Olive Oil
- 3 Cups Vegetable Broth
- 2 Tablespoons Lemon Juice, Fresh
- ½ Teaspoon Garlic Powder
- ½ Cup Carrots, Shredded
- 2 Cups Cabbage, Shredded
- 1 Cup Beets, Shredded
- Dill for Garnish
- ½ Teaspoon Onion Powder
- Sea Salt & Black Pepper to Taste

Directions:

1. Heat oil in a pot, and then sauté your vegetables.
2. Pour your broth in, mixing in your seasoning. Simmer until it's cooked through, and then top with dill.

Nutrition:

Kcal: 263

Carbohydrates: 8 g

Protein: 20.3 g

Fat: 24 g

38. Spinach and Kale Soup

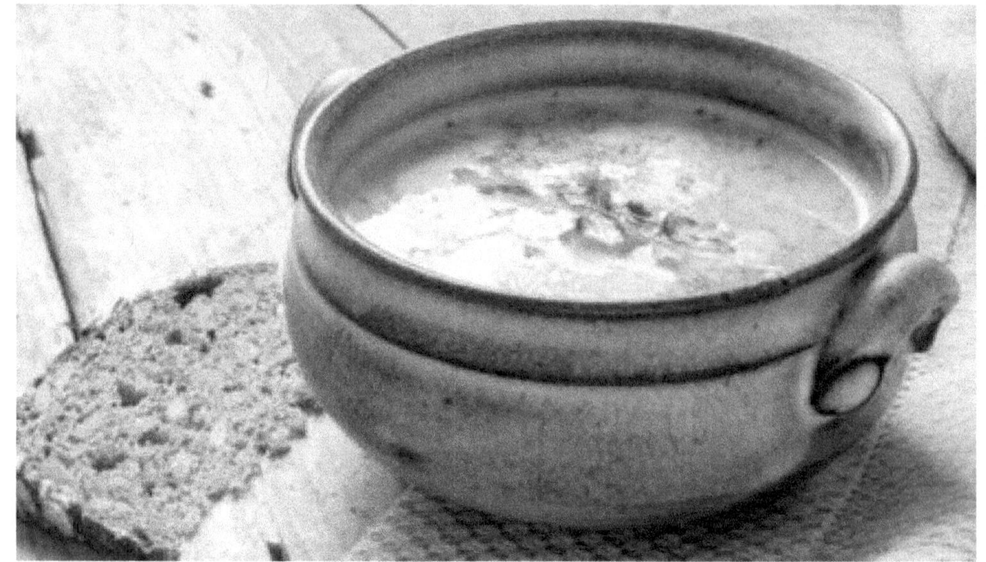

Preparation Time: 5 Minutes

Cooking Time: 5 Minutes

Servings: 2

Ingredients:

- 3 oz. vegan butter
- 1 cup fresh spinach, chopped coarsely
- 1 cup fresh kale, chopped coarsely
- 1 large avocado
- 3 tbsp chopped fresh mint leaves
- 3 ½ cups coconut cream
- 1 cup vegetable broth
- Salt and black pepper to taste
- 1 lime, juiced

Directions:

1. Dissolve the butter in a pot over medium heat and sauté the kale and spinach until wilted, 3 minutes. Turn the heat off.

2. Stir in the remaining ingredients and using an immersion blender, puree the soup until smooth.

3. Dish the soup and serve warm.

Nutrition:

Calories 380

Fat 10 g

Protein 20 g

Carbohydrates 30 g

39. Coconut and Grilled Vegetable Soup

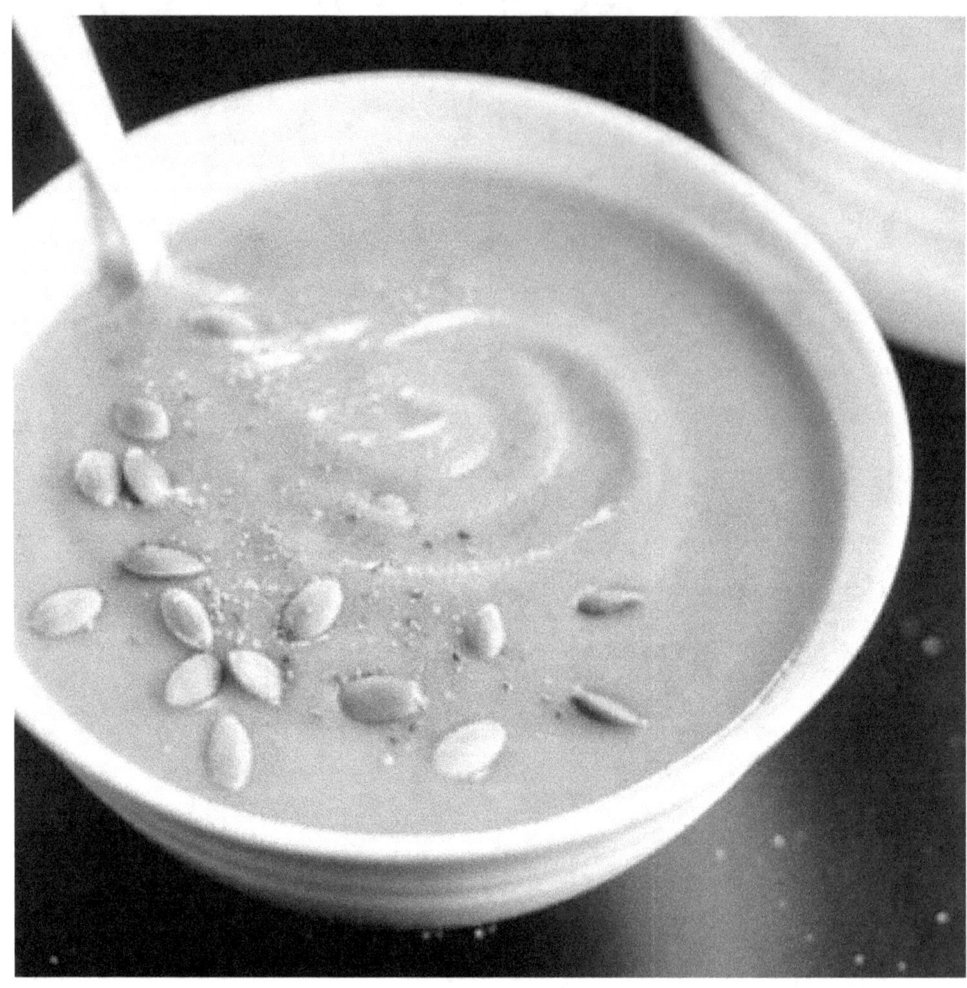

Preparation Time: 10 Minutes

Cooking Time: 45 Minutes

Servings: 4

Ingredients:

- 2 small red onions cut into wedges
- 2 garlic cloves
- 10 oz. butternut squash, peeled and chopped
- 10 oz. pumpkins, peeled and chopped
- 4 tbsp melted vegan butter

- Salt and black pepper to taste
- 1 cup of water
- 1 cup unsweetened coconut milk
- 1 lime juiced
- ¾ cup vegan mayonnaise
- Toasted pumpkin seeds for garnishing

Directions:

1. Preheat the oven to 400 F.
2. On a baking sheet, spread the onions, garlic, butternut squash, and pumpkins and drizzle half of the butter on top. Season with salt, black pepper, and rub the seasoning well onto the vegetables. Roast in the oven for 45 minutes or until the vegetables are golden brown and softened.
3. Transfer the vegetables to a pot; add the remaining ingredients except for the pumpkin seeds and using an immersion blender puree the fixing until smooth.
4. Dish the soup, garnish with the pumpkin seeds and serve warm.

Nutrition:

Calories 290

Fat 10 g

Protein 30 g

Carbohydrates 0 g

40. Broccoli Fennel Soup

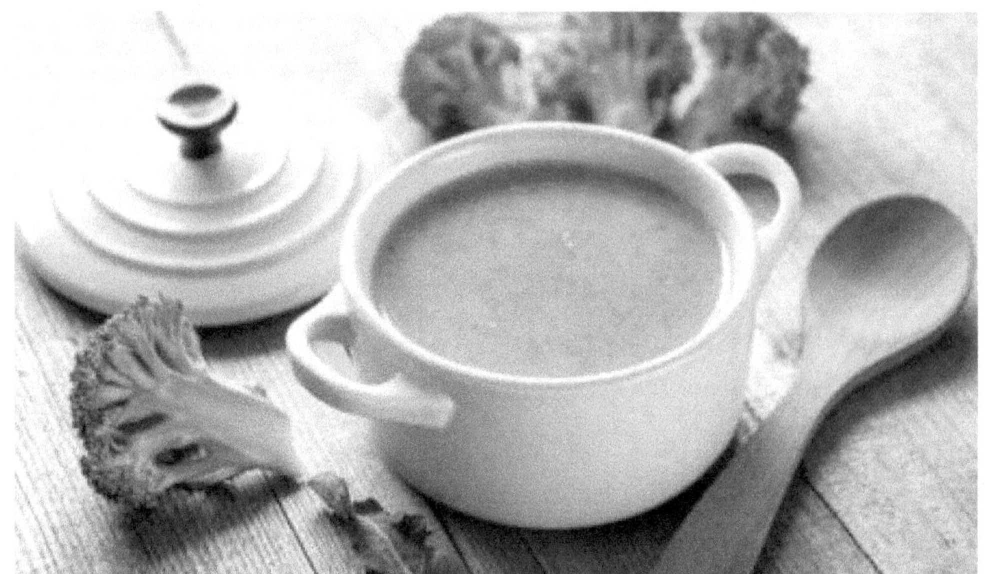

Preparation Time: 15 Minutes

Cooking Time: 10 Minutes

Servings: 4

Ingredients:

- 1 fennel bulb, white and green parts coarsely chopped
- 10 oz. broccoli, cut into florets
- 3 cups vegetable stock
- Salt and freshly ground black pepper
- 1 garlic clove
- 1 cup dairy-free cream cheese
- 3 oz. vegan butter
- ½ cup chopped fresh oregano

Directions:

1. In a medium pot, combine the fennel, broccoli, vegetable stock, salt, and black pepper. Bring to a boil until the vegetables soften, 10 to 15 minutes.
2. Stir in the remaining ingredients and simmer the soup for 3 to 5 minutes.
3. Add salt and black pepper, and dish the soup.

4. Serve warm.

Nutrition:

Calories 240

Fat 0 g

Protein 0 g

Carbohydrates 20 g

41. Pesto Pea Soup

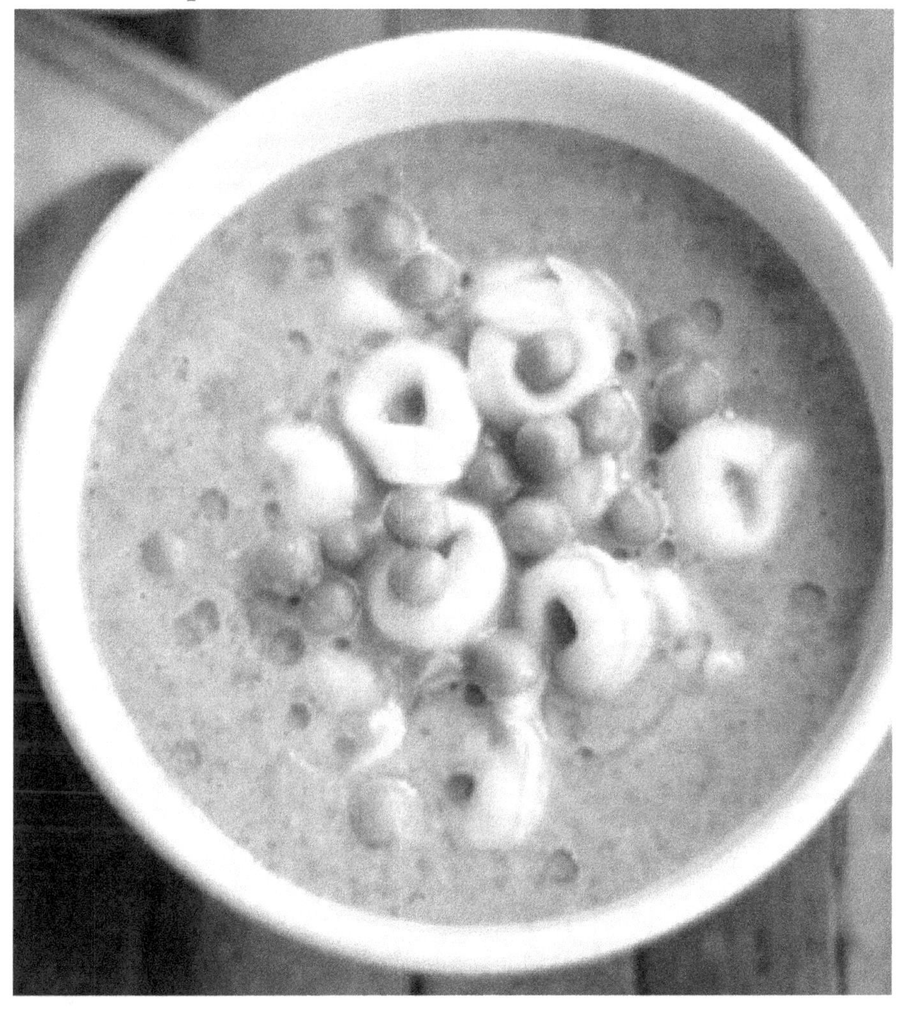

Preparation Time: 10 Minutes

Cooking Time: 20 Minutes

Servings: 4

Ingredients:

- 2 cups Water
- 8 oz. Tortellini
- ¼ cup Pesto
- 1 Onion, small & finely chopped
- 1 lb. Peas, frozen
- 1 Carrot, medium & finely chopped
- 1 ¾ cup Vegetable Broth, less sodium
- 1 Celery Rib, medium & finely chopped

Directions:

1. To start with, boil the water in a large pot over a medium-high heat.
2. Next, stir in the tortellini to the pot and cook it following the instructions given in the packet.
3. In the meantime, cook the onion, celery, and carrot in a deep saucepan along with the water and broth.
4. Cook the celery-onion mixture for 6 minutes or until softened.
5. Now, spoon in the peas and allow it to simmer while keeping it uncovered.
6. Cook the peas for few minutes or until they are bright green and soft.
7. Then, spoon in the pesto to the peas mixture. Combine well.
8. Empty the mixture into a high-speed blender and blend for 2 to 3 minutes or until you get a rich, smooth soup.
9. Return the soup to the pan. Spoon in the cooked tortellini.
10. Finally, pour into a serving bowl and top with more cooked peas if desired.
11. Tip: If desired, you can season it with Maldon salt at the end.

Nutrition:

Calories 100

Fat 0 g

Protein 0 g

Carbohydrates 0 g

42. Tofu and Mushroom Soup

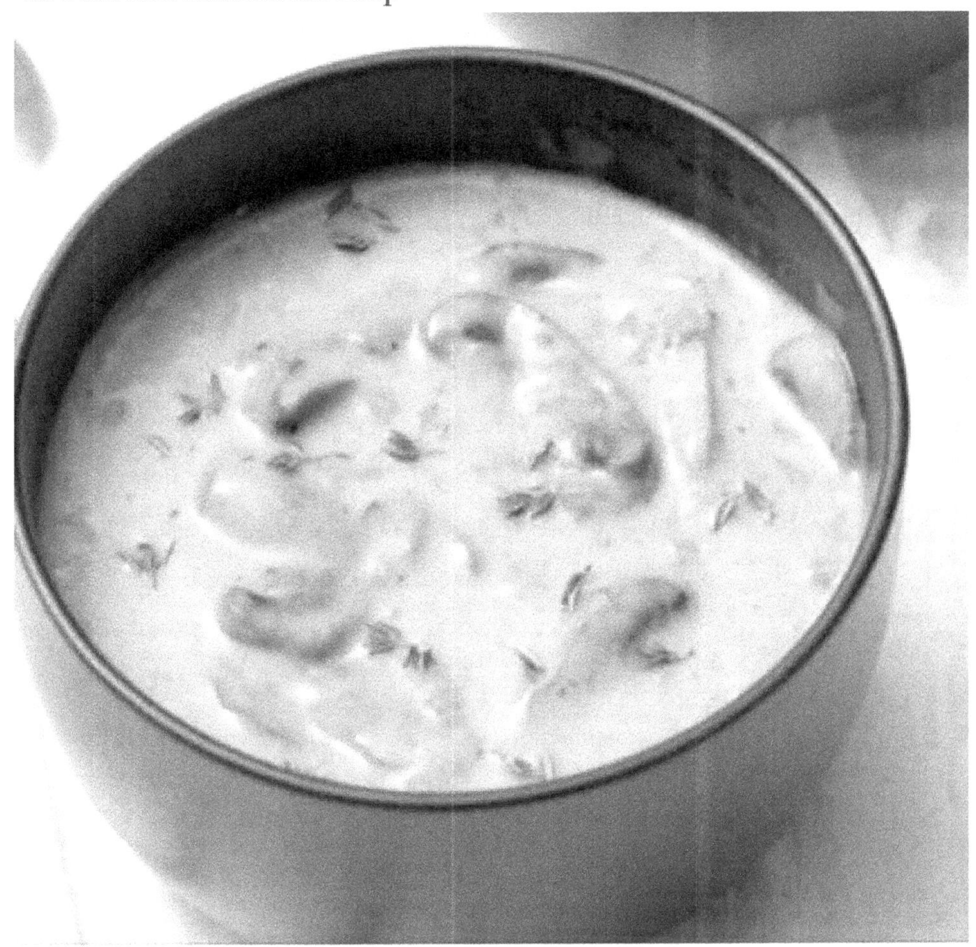

Preparation Time: 15 Minutes

Cooking Time: 10 Minutes

Servings: 4

Ingredients:

- 2 tbsp olive oil
- 1 garlic clove, minced
- 1 large yellow onion, finely chopped
- 1 tsp freshly grated ginger

- 1 cup vegetable stock
- 2 small potatoes, peeled and chopped
- ¼ tsp salt
- ¼ tsp black pepper
- 2 (14 oz) silken tofu, drained and rinsed
- 2/3 cup baby Bella mushrooms, sliced
- 1 tbsp chopped fresh oregano
- 2 tbsp chopped fresh parsley to garnish

Directions:

1. Heat the olive oil in a pan over heat and sauté the garlic, onion, and ginger until soft and fragrant.
2. Pour in the vegetable stock, potatoes, salt, and black pepper. Cook until the potatoes soften, 12 minutes.
3. Stir in the tofu and using an immersion blender, puree the ingredients until smooth.
4. Mix in the mushrooms and simmer with the pot covered until the mushrooms warm up while occasionally stirring to ensure that the tofu doesn't curdle, 7 minutes.
5. Stir oregano, and dish the soup.
6. Garnish with the parsley and serve warm.

Nutrition:

Calories 310

Fat 10 g

Protein 40.0 g

Carbohydrates 0 g

Chapter 10.   Salad and Dessert Recipes

43. Roasted Almond Protein Salad

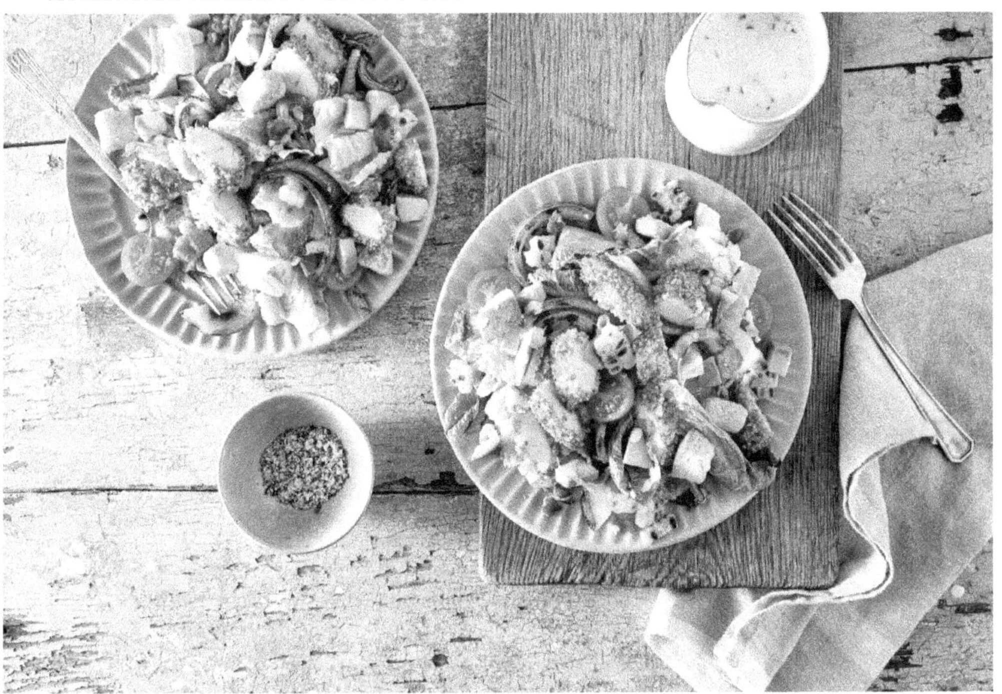

Preparation Time: 30 minutes

Cooking Time: 0 minutes

Servings: 4

Ingredients:

- ½ cup dry quinoa
- ½ cup dry navy beans
- ½ cup dry chickpeas
- ½ cup raw whole almonds
- 1 tsp. extra virgin olive oil
- ½ tsp. salt
- ½ tsp. paprika
- ½ tsp. cayenne
- Dash of chili powder

- 4 cups spinach, fresh or frozen
- ¼ cup purple onion, chopped

Directions:

1. Prepare the quinoa according to the recipe. Store in the fridge for now.
2. Prepare the beans according to the method. Store in the fridge for now.
3. Toss the almonds, olive oil, salt, and spices in a large bowl, and stir until the ingredients are evenly coated.
4. Put a skillet over medium-high heat, and transfer the almond mixture to the heated skillet.
5. Roast while stirring until the almonds are browned, around 5 minutes. You may hear the ingredients pop and crackle in the pan as they warm up. Stir frequently to prevent burning.
6. Put off the heat and toss the cooked and chilled quinoa and beans, onions, and spinach or mixed greens in the skillet. Stir well before transferring the roasted almond salad to a bowl.
7. Enjoy the salad with a dressing of choice, or, store for later!

Nutrition:

Calories 347

Total Fat 10.5g

Sodium 324mg

Protein 17.2g

44. Minty Fruit Salad

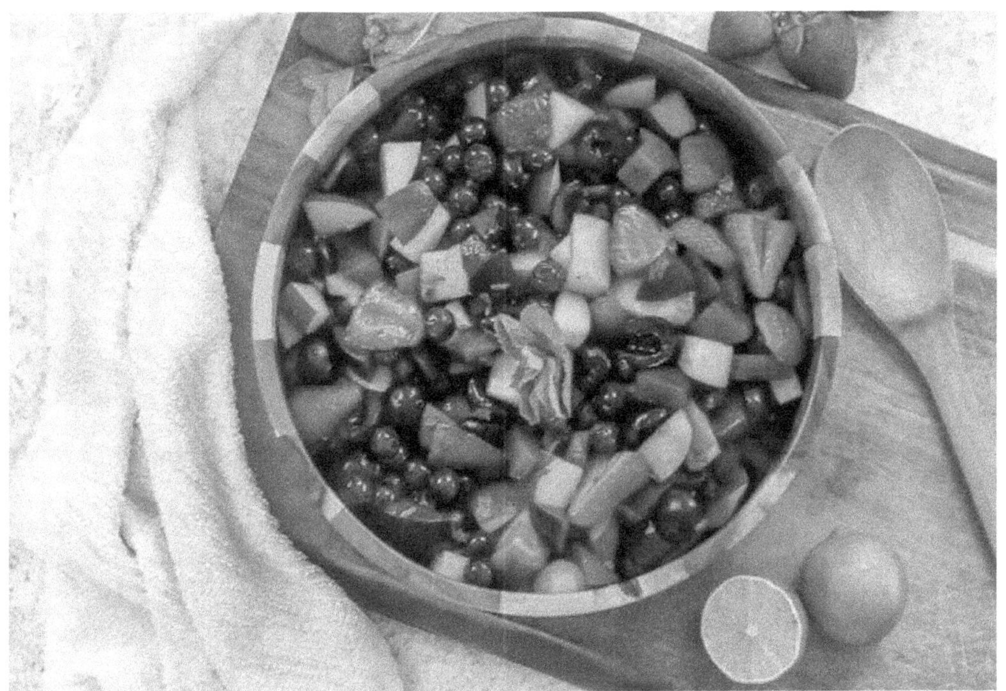

Preparation Time: 15 minutes

Cooking Time: 5 minutes

Servings: 4

Ingredients:

- ¼ cup lemon juice (about 2 small lemons)
- 4 teaspoons maple syrup or agave syrup
- 2 cups chopped pineapple
- 2 cups chopped strawberries
- 2 cups raspberries
- 1 cup blueberries
- 8 fresh mint leaves

Directions:

Preparing the Ingredients.

1. Beginning with 1 mason jar, add the ingredients in this order:

2. 1 tbsp of lemon juice, 1 tsp of maple syrup, ½ cup of pineapple, ½ cup of strawberries, ½ cup of raspberries, ¼ cup of blueberries, and 2 mint leaves.
3. Repeat to fill 3 more jars. Close the jars tightly with lids.
4. Place the airtight jars in the refrigerator for up to 3 days.

Nutrition:

Calories 339

Fat 17.5 g

Carbohydrates 2 g

Sugar 2 g

Protein 44 g

Cholesterol 100 mg

45. Mango Coconut Cream Pie

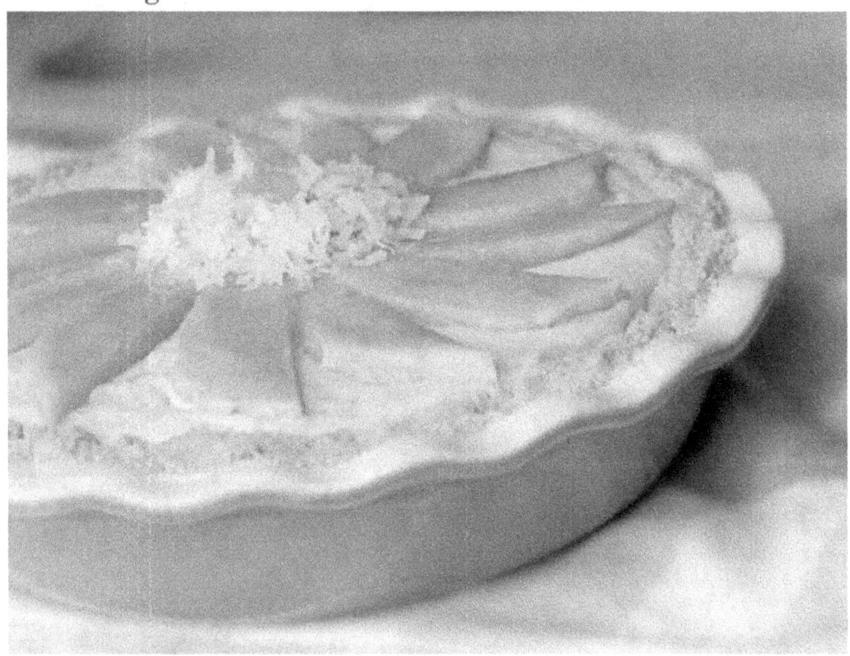

Preparation Time: 20 minutes

Cooking Time: 30 minutes

Servings: 8

Ingredients:

- For the crust
- ½ cup rolled oats
- 1 cup cashews
- 1 cup soft pitted dates
- For the filling
- 1 cup canned coconut milk
- ½ cup water
- 2 large mangos, peeled and chopped, or about 2 cups frozen chunks
- ½ cup unsweetened shredded coconut

Directions:

1. Preparing the Ingredients.
2. Add all the crust ingredients in a food processor and pulse until it holds together. If you don't have a food processor, chop everything as finely as possible and use ½ cup cashew or almond butter in place of half the cashews. Press the mixture down firmly into an 8-inch pie or springform pan.
3. Put the all filling ingredients in a blender and purée until smooth (about 1 minute). It should be very thick, so you may have to stop and stir until it's smooth.
4. Empty the filling into the crust, use a rubber spatula to smooth the top. Once frozen, it should be set out for about 15 minutes to soften before serving.
5. Top with a batch of Coconut Whipped Cream scooped on top of the pie once it's set.

Nutrition:

Calories 545

Fat 39.6 g

Carbohydrates 9.5 g

Sugar 3.1 g

Protein 43 g

Cholesterol 110 mg

46. Lime in the Coconut Chia Pudding

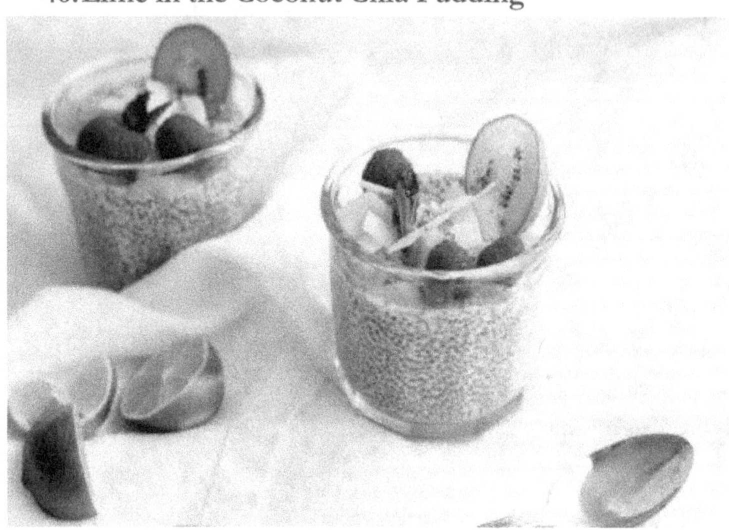

Preparation Time: 10 minutes

Cooking Time: 20 minutes

Servings: 4

Ingredients:

- Zest and juice of 1 lime
- 1 (14-ounce) can coconut milk
- 1 to 2 dates, or 1 tablespoon coconut or other unrefined sugar, or 1 tablespoon maple syrup, or 10 to 15 drops pure liquid stevia
- 2 tablespoons chia seeds, whole or ground
- 2 teaspoons matcha green tea powder (optional)

Directions:

1. Preparing the Ingredients.
2. Grind all the fixings in a blender until smooth. Chill in the fridge for about 20 minutes, then serve topped with one or more of the topping ideas.
3. Try blueberries, blackberries, sliced strawberries, Coconut Whipped Cream, or toasted unsweetened coconut.

Nutrition:

Calories 381

Fat 17.1 g

Carbohydrates 4.1 g

Sugar 0.6 g

Protein 50.6 g

Cholesterol 358 mg

Chapter 11.   Grains and Beans

47. Brown Rice with Mushrooms

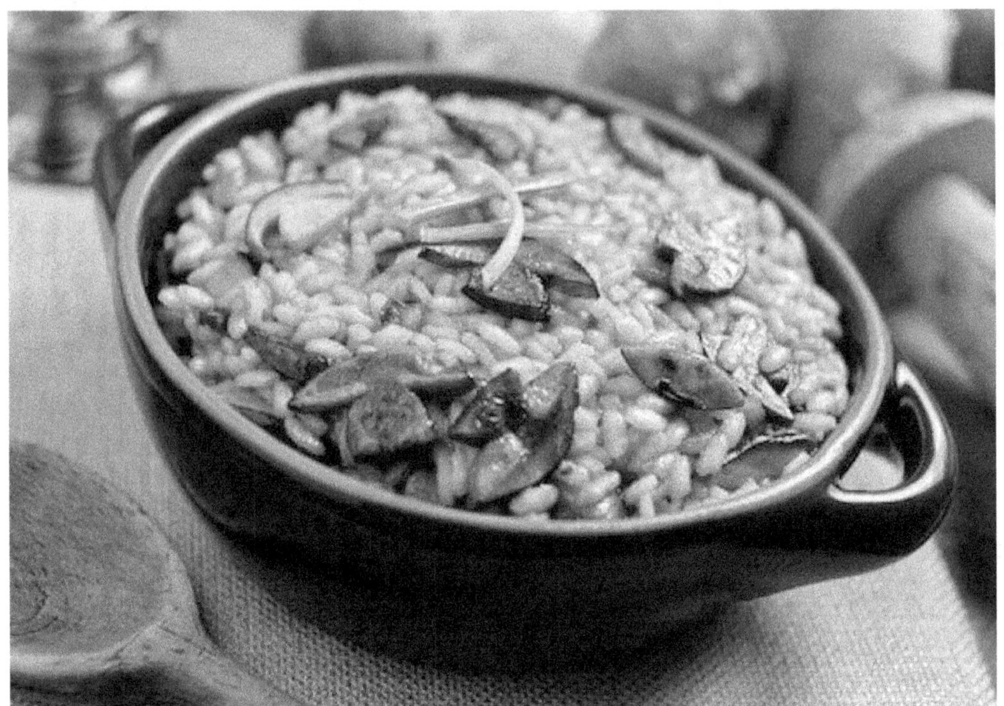

Preparation Time: 15 minutes

Cooking Time: 20 minutes

Servings: 6 to 8

Ingredients:

- ½ pound (227 g) mushrooms, sliced
- 1 green bell pepper, chopped
- 1 onion, chopped
- 1 bunch scallions, chopped
- 2 cloves garlic, minced
- ½ cup water
- 5 cups cooked brown rice
- 1 (16-ounce / 454-g) can chopped tomatoes
- 1 (4-ounce / 113-g) can chopped green chilies
- 2 teaspoons chili powder

- 1 teaspoon ground cumin

Directions:

1. In a large pot, sauté the mushrooms, green pepper, onion, scallions, and garlic in the water for 10 minutes.
2. Stir in the remaining ingredients. Cook over heat for about 10 minutes, or until heated through, stirring frequently.
3. Serve immediately.

Nutrition:

Calories: 185

Fat: 2.6g

Carbs: 34.5g

Protein: 6.1g

Fiber: 4.3g

48. Brown Rice with Spiced Vegetables

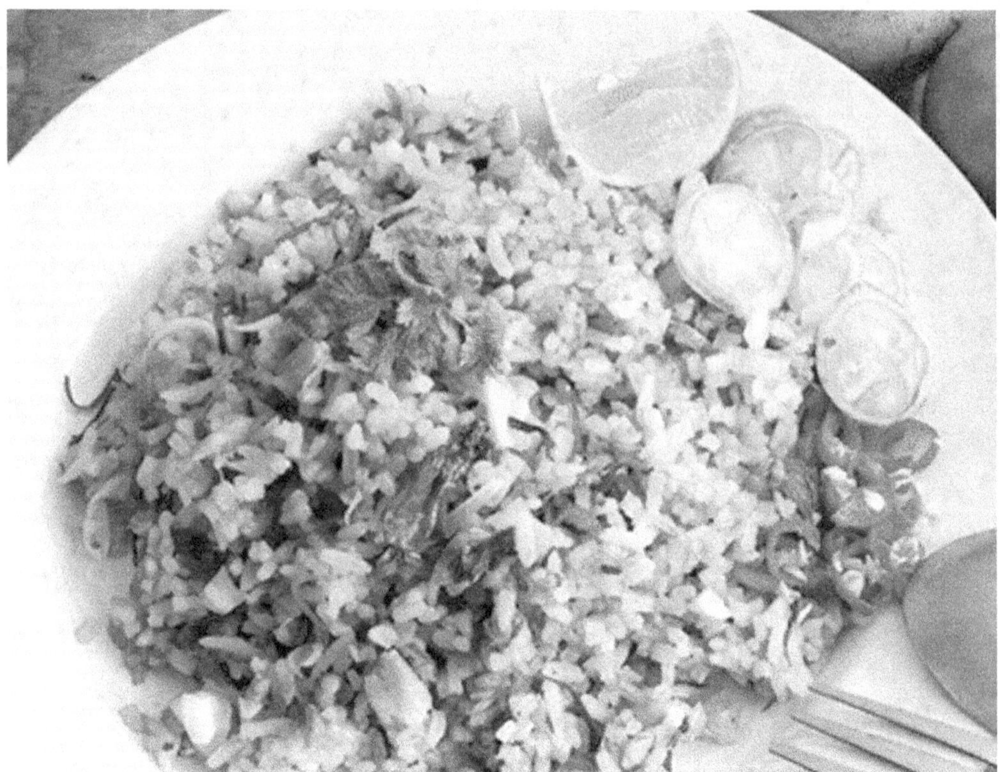

Preparation Time: 10 minutes

Cooking Time: 16 to 18 minutes

Servings: 6

Ingredients:

- 2 teaspoons grated fresh ginger
- 2 cloves garlic, crushed
- ½ cup water
- ¼ pound (113 g) green beans, trimmed and cut into 1-inch pieces
- 1 carrot, scrubbed and sliced
- ½ pound (227 g) mushrooms, sliced
- 2 zucchinis,
- 1 bunch scallions, cut into 1-inch pieces
- 4 cups cooked brown rice
- 3 tablespoons soy sauce

Directions:

1. Place the ginger and garlic in a large pot with the water. Add the green beans and carrot and sauté for 3 minutes.
2. Add the mushrooms and sauté for another 2 minutes. Stir in the zucchini and scallions. Reduce the heat. Cook for 8 minutes, or until the vegetables are tender-crisp, stirring frequently.
3. Stir in the rice and soy sauce. Cook over heat for 5 minutes, or until heated through.
4. Serve warm.

Nutrition:

Calories: 205

Fat: 3.0g

Carbs: 38.0g

Protein: 6.4g

Fiber:4.4 g

49. Black Beans

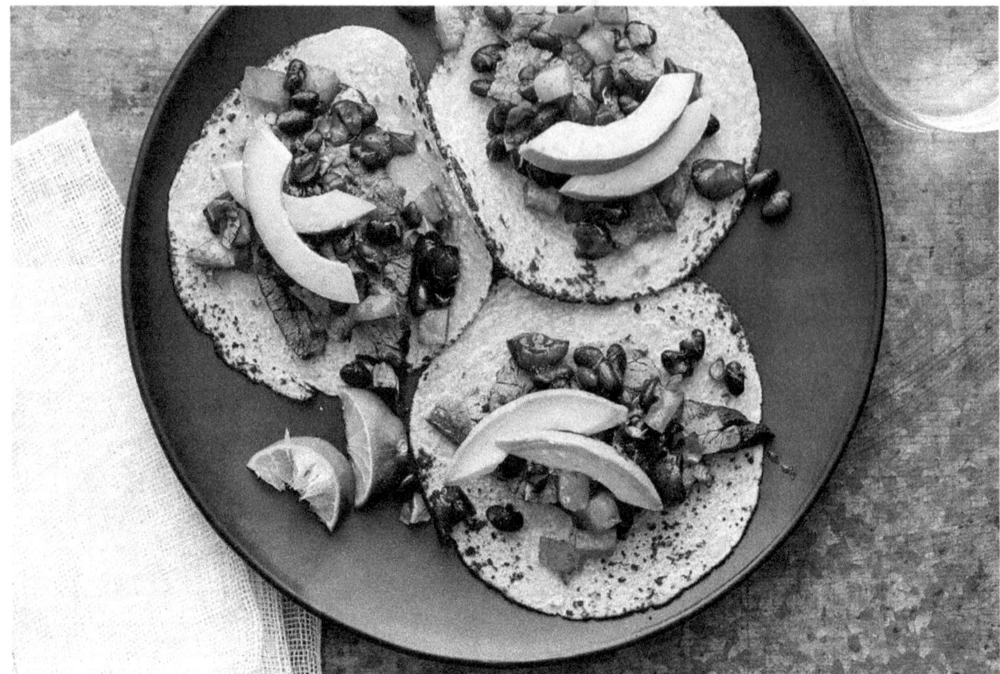

Preparation Time: 10 minutes

Cooking Time: 2 hours

Servings: 8

Ingredients:

- 1 pound (454 g) black beans, soaked overnight and drained
- 10½ cups water, divided
- 1 green bell pepper, cut in half
- 1 onion, finely chopped
- 1 green bell pepper, finely chopped
- 4 cloves garlic, pressed
- 1 tablespoon maple syrup (optional)
- 1 tablespoon Mrs. Dash seasoning
- 1 bay leaf
- ¼ teaspoon dried oregano
- 2 tablespoons cider vinegar

Directions:

1. Place the beans, 10 cups of the water, and green bell pepper in a large pot. Cook over medium heat for about 45 minutes, or until the green pepper is tendered. Remove the green pepper and discard.
2. Meanwhile, in a different pot, combine the onion, chopped green pepper, garlic and the remaining ½ cup of the water. Sauté for 20 minutes
3. Add 1 cup of the cooked beans to the pot with vegetables. Puree the beans and vegetables with a potato masher. Cook over low heat for 1 hour.
4. Drizzle in the vinegar and continue to cook for another hour.
5. Serve warm.

Nutrition:

Calories: 226

Fat: 0.9g

Carbs: 42.7g

Protein: 12.9g

Fiber: 9.9g

50. Noodle and Rice Pilaf

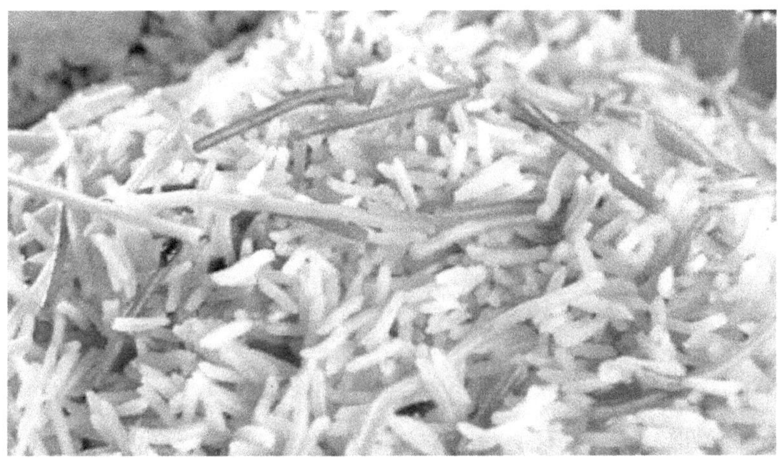

Preparation Time: 5 minutes

Cooking Time: 33 to 44 minutes

Servings: 6 to 8

Ingredients:

- 1 cup whole-wheat noodles, broken into 1/8 inch pieces
- 2 cups long-grain brown rice
- 6½ cups low-sodium vegetable broth
- 1 teaspoon ground cumin
- ½ teaspoon dried oregano

Directions:

1. Combine the noodles and rice in a saucepan over medium heat and cook for 3 to 4 minutes, or until they begin to smell toasted.
2. Stir in the vegetable broth, cumin and oregano. Bring to a boil. Reduce the heat to medium-low. Cook for 40 minutes.

Nutrition:

Calories: 287

Fat: 2.5g

Carbs: 58.1g

Protein: 7.9g

Fiber: 5.0g

51. Spicy Beans and Rice

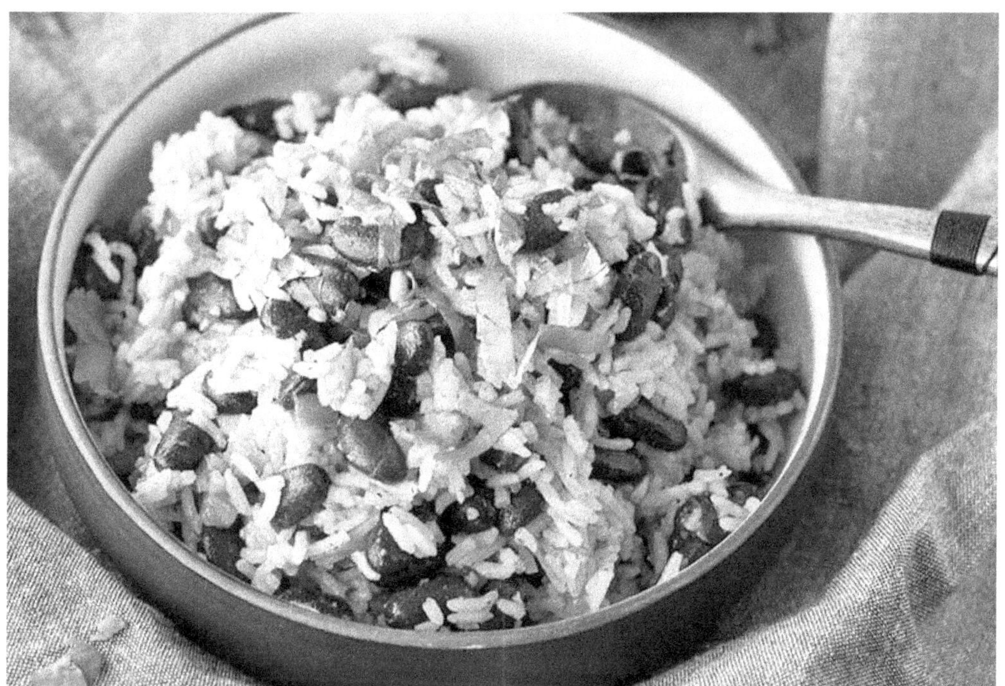

Preparation Time: 5 minutes

Cooking Time: 45 minutes

Servings: 4 to 6

Ingredients:

- 1½ cups long-grain brown rice
- 1 (19-ounce / 539-g) can kidney beans, rinsed and drained
- 2 cups chopped onion
- 1 cup mild salsa
- 1 teaspoon ground cumin
- 16 ounces (454 g) tomatoes, chopped
- 3 cups water

Directions:

1. In a pot, boil water. Stir in the rice. Boil again and stir in the remaining ingredients, except for the tomatoes. Return to a boil. Reduce the heat to low. Cover and simmer for 45 minutes.

2. Remove from the heat and add the tomatoes. Let sit for 5 minutes, covered.

Nutrition:

Calories: 386

Fat: 7.1g

Carbs: 71.1g

Protein: 11.1g

Fiber: 5.8g

Chapter 12.   7 Days Meal Plan

Days	Breakfast	Lunch	Dinner
1	Avocado toast with white beans	chickpea sunflower sandwich	Dijon maple burgers
2	Oatmeal & peanut butter breakfast bar	White bean and artichoke sandwich	Hearty black lentil curry
3	Chocolate chip banana pancake	Egg salad sandwich	Spicy black-eyed peas
4	Avocado and 'sausage' breakfast sandwich	Sabich sandwich	Creamy artichoke soup
5	Vegan variety poppywaw2 seed scones	Tofu and pesto sandwich	Tomato artichoke soup
6	Sweet pomegranate porridge	Chickpea and mayonnaise salad sandwich	Super radish avocado salad
7	Apple oatmeal	Mushrooms sandwich	Beauty school ginger cucumbers

Conclusion

In a nutshell, this cookbook offers you a world full of options to diversify your plant-based menu. People on this diet are usually seen struggling to choose between healthy food and flavor but, soon, they run out of the options. The selection of the recipes in this book is enough to adorn your table with flavorsome, plant-based meals every day. Give each recipe a good read and try them out in the kitchen. You will experience tempting aromas and binding flavors every day.

The book is conceptualized with the idea of offering you a comprehensive view of a plant-based diet and how it can benefit the body. You may find the shift sudden, especially if you are a die-hard fan of non-vegetarian items. But you need not give up anything that you love. Eat everything in moderation.

The next step is to start experimenting with the different recipes in this book and see which ones are your favorites. Everyone has their favorite food, and you will surely find several of yours in this book. Begin with breakfast and work your way through. You will be pleasantly surprised at how tasty a vegan meal really can be.

Now you have what you need to start making budget-friendly, healthy plant-based recipes. Just follow your basic shopping list and follow your meal plan to get started! It's easy to switch over to a plant-based diet if you have your meals planned out and temptation locked away. Don't forget to clean out your kitchen before starting, and you're sure to meet all your diet and health goals.

If dieting seems very important to you and you need to do it right, then it is recommended that you visit a professional such as a nutritionist or dietitian to discuss your dieting plan and optimizing it for the better.

No matter how much you want to lose weight, it is not advised that you decrease your calorie intake to an unhealthy level. Losing weight does not mean that you stop eating. It is done by carefully planning meals.

A plant-based diet is very easy once you get into it. At first, you will start to face a lot of difficulties, but if you start slowly, then you can face all the barriers and achieve your goal.

Swap out one unhealthy food item each week that you know is not helping you and put in its place one of the plant-based ingredients that you like. Then have some fun creating the many different recipes in this book. Find out what recipes you like the most so you can make them often and most of all; have some fun exploring all your recipe options.

Wish you good luck with the plant-based diet!